How to Develop Your Healthcare Career

A Guide to Employability and Professional Development

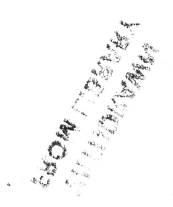

How to Develop Your Healthcare Career

A Guide to Employability and Professional Development

Edited by

Lisa Taylor

Occupational Therapy Lecturer
University of East Anglia

WILEY Blackwell   BMJ|Books

This edition first published 2016 © 2016 by John Wiley & Sons, Ltd

BMJ Books is an imprint of BMJ Publishing Group Limited, used under licence by John Wiley & Sons.

Registered Office
John Wiley & Sons, Ltd, The Atrium, Southern Gate, Chichester, West Sussex, PO19 8SQ, UK

Editorial Offices
9600 Garsington Road, Oxford, OX4 2DQ, UK
The Atrium, Southern Gate, Chichester, West Sussex, PO19 8SQ, UK
111 River Street, Hoboken, NJ 07030-5774, USA

For details of our global editorial offices, for customer services and for information about how to apply for permission to reuse the copyright material in this book please see our website at www.wiley.com/wiley-blackwell

Library of Congress Cataloging-in-Publication data applied for

ISBN: 9781118910832

A catalogue record for this book is available from the British Library.

Wiley also publishes its books in a variety of electronic formats. Some content that appears in print may not be available in electronic books.

Cover image: Meaden Creative

Set in 9.5/12pt Minion by SPi Global, Pondicherry, India
Printed in Singapore by C.O.S. Printers Pte Ltd

1   2016

Contents

Contributors

Stephanie Allen
Leadership skills facilitator and coach, The Training Spa, Norwich, UK

David Dowdeswell-Allaway
Freelance writer, trainer and facilitator, Norwich, UK

Professor James Gazzard
Associate Dean for Postgraduate Taught Courses, Enterprise and Engagement, School of Health Sciences, Faculty of Medicine and Health Sciences, University of East Anglia, Norwich, UK

Adrienne Jolly
Careers Adviser (Arts & Humanities), Career Service, University of East Anglia, Norwich, UK

Jonathan Larner
Physiotherapy Course Director, School of Health Sciences, University of East Anglia, Norwich, UK

Dr Rosemarie Mason
Course Director for BSc in Occupational Therapy, School of Health Sciences, University of East Anglia, Norwich, UK

Neil Sellen
Leadership & OD Team, Health Education East of England, Fulbourn, Cambridge, UK

Dr Lisa Taylor
Occupational Therapy Lecturer & Academic Employability Lead, School of Health Sciences, University of East Anglia, Norwich, UK

Foreword

Not long after I qualified as a physiotherapist, I began to realise that I needed to do more than simply hone and develop my clinical skills if I was to be successful in my vocation – that being simply to make a difference to people's lives. It wasn't about ambition or success, it was about employability. If only this book had been available to me then, I would have been able to focus more quickly on what I needed to do!

A number of phrases stand out when reading this book: 'personal responsibility' and 'going the extra mile'. Being a professional healthcare clinician is so much more than clinical competence and this book takes you through what you need to develop in order to become a well-rounded professional – even exploring what being professional means – all of which makes you more employable. I would particularly draw your attention to the chapter on business skills, simply because it is quite possibly the section that you will feel less inclined to read or that you feel has less relevance to health care. In fact, the opposite is true! I have interviewed hundreds of clinicians of all tribes for jobs over my career and these business skills are definitely what are more and more sought after today.

On a more basic level, understanding the healthcare context in which you are working is vital to ensuring that what you are doing is relevant and will make the difference you want. As you start your career, appreciating that you will not be working in a vacuum shows a level of maturity – and makes you more employable!

All of the above, and more, require you taking personal responsibility – no one else can do this for you. You cannot expect others to nurture and develop you if you do not do it for yourself and this does require additional effort.

This brings me to the second point of 'going the extra mile'. If you want to be more employable, this is what you will need to do – do that bit more – and it is an investment that will pay dividends in the long run. People talk about those that are successful as being 'lucky'. I believe you make your own luck and this book gives you a brilliant framework for just doing a bit more to develop into a successful, rounded clinician who will get noticed and become 'lucky'!

I sincerely commend this book to you and really only wish that it had been available to me at the beginning of my clinical career but also at numerous points on my journey when I felt stuck.

Professor Karen Middleton, CBE
Chief Executive, Chartered Society of Physiotherapy (CSP)

Karen Middleton has been a regular commentator on health policy and before her current position was chief health professions officer at NHS England and the Department of Health – the Government's most senior adviser on the allied health professions.

Preface

Many students may go through their university education without a thought about their employability. The lack of attention paid to employability is surprising given the changing health and social care environment that graduates will be entering, wherever they are in the world. Awareness of employability is key in preparing and evidencing what you have to offer employing organisations. Employability awareness is of crucial importance throughout education if healthcare graduates are to maximise their employment potential. Individuals need to ensure that they keep abreast of the requirements and opportunities within the world of work as the health and social care environment is constantly changing. Ill prepared graduates are less likely to be able to provide evidence or be able to confidently articulate their employability when it comes to applying for jobs. To our knowledge this is the first book that provides you with key topics relating to healthcare employability in one book. The style of the book encourages you to embark on a personal journey of employability – reflecting and acting upon the knowledge that you have acquired. Having read and engaged with the content of this book you will have generated evidence and confidence to articulate your employability.

What is employability?

Trying to answer the question of 'What is Employability?' continues to throw up as many questions as it answers! A discussion of the history and concept of employability is presented in the first chapter of this book. But, in essence:

- *Employability* is the *process* of equipping yourself to be able to apply for and fulfil the personal specifications of a job.
- *Employment* is the *successful outcome* of you evidencing and articulating your employability through the job recruitment process.

Who should read this book?

Employability is a lifelong journey and although this book is predominantly targeted at healthcare pre-registration students and early career healthcare professionals, the guiding principles delivered within it are relevant for many healthcare practitioners, however far along their employability journey they are. Additionally, those involved with healthcare education will find the information presented useful to support and facilitate the development of their student's employability. Many of the contextual examples in this book relate to the United Kingdom but the principles are transferable for health professionals regardless of where they are working in the world.

Why read this book?

This book will provide you with information on topics that are most pertinent to enhance your employability. It will give you time to consider where you are and where you want to be in relation to your employability, which will be crucial in determining your career path. There is the opportunity for reflection as you read each chapter, so that the book becomes a handbook of employability that you can work through individually to maximise your employability potential. Suggested interview questions are posed at the end of each chapter for your consideration. The final chapter in the book provides an opportunity for you to consolidate your learning through a series of activities.

How to use this book

This book is divided into a number of chapters relating to key aspects of employability:

- *Chapter 1 What is employability and what does it mean for you?* – providing the theory underpinning the continuing debate about graduate employability and what the theory means for you in practice.
- *Chapter 2 Career planning and management* – an opportunity to consider what a career is and what it means to you, and how you can influence your career by the choices that you make.
- *Chapter 3 Professionalism* – a thorough exploration of professionalism as a concept and your individual responsibility to uphold professionalism within your work.
- *Chapter 4 Continuing professional development* – as an essential part of demonstrating employability – the concept and practice of continuing professional development is discussed.

- *Chapter 5 Leadership* – presents types of leadership that will be practised by all healthcare practitioners and considers higher level aspirational leadership opportunities.
- *Chapter 6 Service improvement* – this area of work is key within a changing health and social care environment and these skills are critical to enhance your employability.
- *Chapter 7 Business skills* – provides an explanation of setting up your own business in an easy to digest format with part of the chapter being focused on social enterprise.
- *Chapter 8 The job application process* – a step by step approach to applying for a job and the main points to consider.
- *Chapter 9 Consolidation of learning and moving forward* – gives you the opportunity to work through a number of activities related to the information presented within each chapter of the book; it is a chance for you to revise the key points and develop some evidence of learning related to each chapter to be used in your continuing professional development portfolio.

It is hoped that you will find this book useful in your employability journey – at whatever stage you are and in whatever environment you are planning to or are working within. The reflections as you read and the consolidation of your learning through the activities provided in the final chapter will provide you with the evidence and confidence to articulate your own employability.

Lisa Taylor
University of East Anglia

Chapter 1 What is employability and what does it mean for you?

Lisa Taylor

School of Health Sciences, University of East Anglia, Norwich, UK

Introduction

Employability may be something that you have never really considered in detail before. Perhaps you have been focusing on completing your studies without really thinking about what will happen when you have finished? Will you continue studying as a postgraduate, go travelling or try to find a job in your chosen profession? Your consideration of your own employability should start as soon as possible and is a lifelong journey of learning and reflection about yourself and what you can offer the world of work. What can the world of work offer you? In a changing health and social care environment the opportunities within your profession are changing too – What do you need to do to respond to that in a proactive manner?

This chapter provides you with some of the history and theory behind employability and encourages you to consider where you are in your employability journey. There are suggestions on what you can do to help develop your own employability. The remainder of the book builds upon the concept of employability presented in this chapter, focusing on key areas of personal and professional development that are particularly relevant for healthcare employability. Throughout this chapter you are encouraged to reflect and consider how the information presented affects you own perceptions of employability and your own employability journey.

Time for reflection

What do you think employability is? How have you considered employability so far in your life? How do you think employability is different to employment?

How to Develop Your Healthcare Career: A Guide to Employability and Professional Development, First Edition. Edited by Lisa Taylor.
© 2016 John Wiley & Sons, Ltd. Published 2016 by John Wiley & Sons, Ltd.

What does the literature say on employability and how it has evolved?

Employability is complex and it is clear from the available literature that being able to develop a precise and clear focus on it as a concept is difficult (Harvey, 2001; Hillage and Pollard, 1998). Employability and career development are very often conflated as concepts but are addressed individually in this book. The debate on employability has been longstanding, reaching far beyond the United Kingdom (Harvey and Knight, 2003). Although the meaning of employability has changed over time (Moreau and Leathwood, 2006), the importance of employability within the strategic direction of the Department of Education has been highlighted (Hillage and Pollard, 1998). Some authors state that employability has historically been viewed from a number of perspectives – economic social, organisational and individual – with the individual perspective emerging more in the 1990s (Nauta et al., 2009).

Rosenburg, Heimler and Morote (2012) discuss employability as the basic skills needed for job performance and once an individual is in employment, employability develops into transferable core proficiencies. They are, therefore, suggesting that employability is a continuing process of personal and professional development. Yorke (2006) states that employability as a concept was developed within education and focuses on the possession of relevant achievements and the ability to function in a job, not actually the process of acquiring a job. Dacre Pool and Sewell (2007) support this assertion, suggesting that employability is more than just getting a job. Employability is rarely defined as an individual being equipped to do a job (Harvey, 2001). Some approaches appear to confuse employability and employment (McQuaid and Lindsay, 2005). Harvey and Knight (2003) present different perspectives on employability – from developing attributes for graduate employment to the ability of a graduate to get a job and to succeed in a job. Therefore, there are a wide range of perspectives on employability, most of which reinforce the notion that employability is more than just a set of skills and is a continuing process.

Time for reflection

How does the literature above inform your understanding of employability as a concept? What and who do you think influences your own employability?

Towards a common language of employability

Despite the arguments presented that propose that employability is wider than just a group of skills that individuals develop, skill acquisition still appears to be the basis used for policy formation (Holmes, 2001). There appears to be an assumption that skills are synonymous with employability (Holmes, 2006). It is critical that education establishments and employers have the same understanding of employability (Holmes, 2001). This shared understanding is essential to ensure consistency in expectations and to assist the transitions individuals make, firstly from studies to employment and then within their careers. It is unfortunate that little research exists to underpin the alternative approaches to the skills approach to employability (Hinchliffe and Jolly, 2011). With employability being high on some governments' agenda (Moreau and Leathwood, 2006), it is crucial that this concept is adequately defined and researched to enable individuals to understand and enhance their employability through a common language.

It is the employers that convert the employability of graduates into employment (Harvey, 2001) – so, as previously suggested, employability is the process of equipping yourself for a job with employment being the outcome when you are actually in a job. You need an awareness of what employers are looking for; this may change in response to policy changes and economic changes, which are critical to keep abreast of. Professional bodies keep abreast and inform members of changes that impact on their profession. However, on a local level the individual needs to understand the impact of changes on the work context. For example, a speech and language service going through the tendering and contracting process requires flexibility and proactiveness of its employees. The journey of employability continues for an individual as he/she continues to develop personally and professionally in their job/s as they develop their careers (Figure 1.1).

Time for reflection

If you could design a model of employability – what would it look like?

Models of employability

The main models of employability reported in the literature are presented here. This provides an opportunity for you to consider how these reflect your understanding of employability and whether they are models that you would find helpful to apply to your own personal construct of employability.

Bennett *et al.* model on course provision

Bennett, Dunne and Carré (1999) proposed a model focusing on course provision within education – with five main areas of focus for education establishments to adequately prepare students for the world of work:

1. Disciplinary content knowledge, for example anatomy and physiology.
2. Disciplinary skills, for example taking someone's blood pressure.
3. Workplace awareness, for example knowledge of what is offered and what is required of you within the hospital workplace or area that you are working.

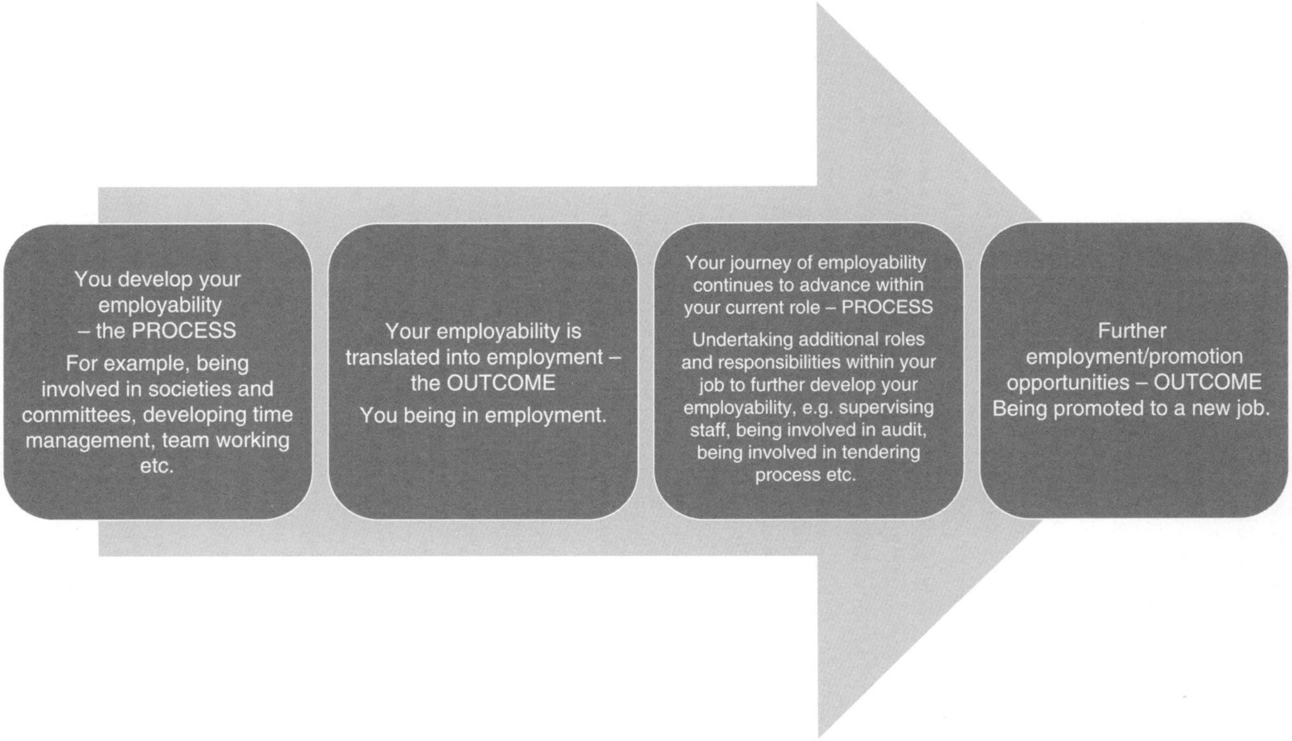

Figure 1.1 The journey of employability

You develop your employability – the PROCESS

For example, being involved in societies and committees, developing time management, team working etc.

Your employability is translated into employment – the OUTCOME You being in employment.

Your journey of employability continues to advance within your current role – PROCESS

Undertaking additional roles and responsibilities within your job to further develop your employability, e.g. supervising staff, being involved in audit, being involved in tendering process etc.

Further employment/promotion opportunities – OUTCOME Being promoted to a new job.

4. Workplace experience, for example placement experiences.
5. Generic skill, for example team working, time management, communication.

Watts DOTS model

Further suggested models include the DOTS model, which is discussed by Watts (2006). It is made up of four main components that break down employability into manageable areas to focus on – *D*ecision learning, *O*pportunity awareness, *T*ransition learning and *S*elf-awareness. The interesting aspect of the DOTS model is a self-awareness of your skills interests and values. For example – if you are a physiotherapist – does women's health interest you or does musculoskeletal physiotherapy interest you? If you are considering working within a social enterprise, do their care values match your values and if they do not match up then how comfortable are you working within such an environment?

Dacre Pool and Sewell Career EDGE model

Career EGDE was presented in a paper by Dacre Pool and Sewell (2007). It is a three-tiered system. In the first tier, the following employability components are included: career development, experience in life and work, degree (knowledge and understanding), generic transferable skills and emotional intelligence to motivate yourself and others. The second tier of the model is a reflection and evaluation tier – reinforcing the importance for you to reflect upon your experiences. The reflection and evaluation feeds into the third tier, which includes self-esteem, self-confidence and self-efficacy. Reflection upon your experiences is something that as healthcare students/practitioners you are used to undertaking regularly.

The unique value of the Career EDGE model lies in its transferability to any stage in a career. It is not exclusive to students, which reinforces the message that employability is a life-long journey and does not end when employment has been secured.

Yorke and Knight USEM model

The USEM (understanding, skills, efficacy beliefs and metacognition) model presented by Yorke and Knight (2006) is reported to be one of the most used and respected models of employability and offers another model that looks beyond the skill development aspect of employability (Hinchliffe and Jolly, 2011; Dacre Pool and Sewell, 2007). The USEM model contributes to a large body of academic work on employability which can make it inaccessible for individuals to use, resulting in it becoming more of a guide for curriculum development rather than a clear guide for personal employability development.

Personal responsibility for employability

What is interesting to note about the models presented is that they reflect that employability is more than just skill development and begin to articulate the importance of self-reflection and awareness. Employability is not something that is undertaken by others for you, it is something that you need to consider and undertake for yourself. If you do not take ownership you risk restricting your personal and professional development, thereby potentially adversely influencing your long-term potential within the world of work. This suggestion of ownership and individual employability identity is supported by evidence reported in the literature. Hinchliffe and Jolly (2011) undertook research to provide some evidence about employer expectations of graduates. A questionnaire was distributed to employers to judge graduate performance and four strands of themes were identified from the research; these are summarised here:

1. *Values* – personal ethics, social and organisation values, including the value associated with entrepreneurship.
2. *Intellect* – how a graduate is able to think critically, to analyse information and to bring about change within organisations.
3. *Performance* – the transfer of skills and ability to learn new skills relevant to the workplace.
4. *Engagement with others* – the ability for graduates to engage with a wide range of challenges and individuals/organisations.

These four strands emphasise the importance of you taking ownership and influencing your own employability, whether it be in response to your own personal values or your motivation to think critically and influence, which could have a positive impact within the working environment. Some of the changes that are happening within health and social care may be difficult to deal with, but employers need individuals who can continue to develop personally and professionally within the working environment despite difficult demands.

Time for reflection

How do your personal values and beliefs influence your focus on employability?

External influences on employability

The limitations of the models presented thus far is that they do not explicitly consider external influences, such as economic, environmental, social or political contexts, that may influence your employability. This is a very real issue within the health and social care sector and something that impacts on career development and planning, as discussed in Chapter 2.

It needs to be acknowledged that external influences, such as economic social and health priorities and policies, will have an influence on your employment options. You need to respond to this to maximise your employability. This is the drawback on focusing purely on skill development rather than taking a holistic approach to employability. You could spend your time developing a specific skill but if, in the meantime, the political landscape has changed there may be different priorities that render your skill worthless. McQuaid and Lindsay (2005) presented seven operational versions of the concept of employability: dichotomic employability; sociomedical employability; manpower policy employability; flow employability; labour market performance and employability; initiative employability; interactive employability. These seven versions of the concept of employability support the suggestion that is not just the individual who influences their own employability – there are external contributory factors that will have an influence on the employability of individuals. There is a concern that there is a perceived narrow concept of employability adopted by policymakers and researchers that does not take into account the personal circumstances and external factors that may influence an individual's employability (McQuaid and Lindsay, 2005). Further literature (Hillage and Pollard, 1998) supports the assertion by McQuaid and Lindsay and presents four components to employability, which include assets, deployment, presentation and also take into account the external influences. External influences could be, for example, government policy changes that result in a change in clinical priorities or changes in family circumstances that restrict an individual's ability to commit to a leadership course that would be useful for employability development.

Time for reflection
What market conditions do you need to be aware of within current health and social care that may influence your employability?

Response to changing expectations within the workplace and personal circumstances

To fully embrace the concept of employability you need to have an awareness of the world of work into which you are entering. Workplace environments are changing and this is no less evident than in the area of health and social care. A psychosocial construct of employability has been presented by Fugate, Kinicki and Ashforth (2004). It identifies that a number of person-centred constructs are required in order to maximise employability and respond to the changing workplace. Fugate, Kinicki and Ashforth (2004) argue that there are three main elements to employability that all have a mutual influence on each other:

1. Career identity.
2. Personal adaptability.
3. Social (networks) and human capital (education and experience).

You need to be increasingly flexible within the modern workplace to adapt to what the job requires you to do. The roles and responsibilities of health professionals are shifting; for example, the introduction of prescribing of medication and injection therapies for nurses and physiotherapists or the setting up of social enterprises to provide health and social care. This means that you may have to change your identity at work multiple times over a period of employment, depending on the demands within your job. The ability for you to adapt to change will be key to your success. This means that past learning needs to be adaptable to new working situations – and this needs to be evidenced to demonstrate this to future employers. For example, if you have been involved in an activity at university that has demonstrated your ability to be flexible and proactive, then use that as an example which is transferable to the work situation. The concept of an internal locus of control is an interesting concept relevant to this situation, whereby your response to external influences will have an impact on the outcome of the situation (Fugate, Kinicki and Ashforth, 2004). There may be external influences on job prospects and changing roles but your individual response to the situation – being optimistic and opportunistic about situations – will maximise your development and opportunities as an individual. Personal circumstances that may have an impact on your employability and response to work situations can also change, such a buying a house in a specific location. In order to maximise your employability potential, an appreciation and awareness of external and personal factors that impact on employability is essential if you are to establish and evidence where you are and how you are able to adapt and respond to the changes.

Time for reflection

How can you ensure that you respond in a proactive manner to change to maximise your opportunities?

A number of models have been presented that have attempted to incorporate the different definitions of employability within a workable model to try to increase the clarity of employability in practice. However, it has been argued that the models presented have been either too complex or too simple (Dacre Pool and Sewell, 2007). The literature does present a wide range of considerations for employability which can inform the development of a personal construct of employability relevant to you.

Time for reflection
Having read the models presented above, does this influence your own personal construct of employability? What model is best applied to your own circumstances?

How is employability approached within education?

Time for reflection
How has employability been addressed within your education?

It is important to consider how employability is approached within education in order to understand the dynamics between education and employability and the potential impact on students. An example of this is presented in Chapter 3 relating to the University of East Anglia (UEA) professionalism charter. Enhancing graduate employability has been part of a wider UK government policy strategy (Harvey, 2000) and does assume a priority within education (Yorke, 2006). It is recognised that subject discipline achievements, such as core clinical skills, are important but it is equally as important to demonstrate achievements outside of a student's subject discipline (Yorke, 2006), such as extracurricular clubs, volunteering and committees and so on. Higher education institutions need to contribute to student employability in a comprehensive manner and not be limited to focusing on specific skills or work experience (Atkins, 1999). However, the focus of employability still remains with skills and attributes (Holmes, 2006) rather than using a holistic approach. Despite attempts to recognise the importance of experiences outside of the degree programme with the introduction of the Higher Education Achievement Report (Pegg et al., 2012), employability does not appear to be fully embraced by staff or students. You need to engage with the concept of employability very early on in your education careers in order to maximise your employability potential. Academics need to be made aware of the importance of employability and the relationship that it has with the curriculum and potential employment.

Within a competitive work market place, employment is not guaranteed (Holmes, 2006) and you need to focus on producing evidence to demonstrate your employability. The focus on education establishments for employability tends to be on the performance league tables, which measure the first destination of graduate employment at six months post-graduation (Smith, McKnight and Naylor, 2000). The focus on employment post-graduation when referring to employability reinforces the confusion between the concepts of employability and employment. The performance league tables are actually measuring employment rather than employability – as we have already ascertained, there is a difference between the two concepts. The performance league tables are important in influencing whether a student will decide to apply to study at a particular university. However, employability is about more than determining consumer choice, despite this being of increasing interest to students and their parents (Maher, 2011). There is a concern that this focus on performance league tables distracts academics from the importance of employability throughout your studies – as purely an outcome rather than a process concept. The role of academics in the development of employability within the curriculum is essential for it to be truly embedded within the university experience, rather than being tagged onto the end of your university experience, when employment becomes the focus for students. Therefore, although you need to take ownership of your own employability, it essential that there is an understanding and support from academic staff as to the importance and application of employability in your student experience from day one.

Some institutions have attempted to assist academics in the translation of employability within the curriculum. The UCLan employability framework (Day, 2009) provides a tool for all of those involved in student education, breaking down employability into 14 areas. These areas have all been allocated a code and are used to badge material presented to students. This system of badging the material that students are exposed to reinforces and highlights employability within the curriculum for students and academics. Employability should be part of the language of students and academics, and the use of employability frameworks is useful in focusing attention and provides a common language for students and academics to use, thereby making employability an explicit part of the student experience. The implementation of employability frameworks within the curriculum does not need to impact on the subject-specific learning but provides some indication on how that learning can evidence a student's employability and translate into the world of work.

It does need to be recognised that a single model of employability, such as the UCLan framework, may not be relevant for all universities, and that there are a number of variables that influence embedding employability within the curriculum (Yorke and Knight, 2006). What universities can do, though, is to take the principles of employability models to apply within their own situations. Engagement of students and academics is key in the process, which has been shown to be problematic in the past (Higher Education Academy, 2012). Clarity in the importance and concepts of employability is key in there being buy-in from already busy academics and students who may not see employability as a priority, to increase engagement and ownership, which is critical for true embedding of employability (Graves, 2011). Realistically, though, the acceptance and application of the concept of employability into everyday life and language is likely to take time for academics and students to adopt (Harvey and Knight, 2003).

Time for reflection

What can you do to make sure that you engage fully with the concept of employability during your studies? What feedback can you provide to your education institution for it to adopt an employability focused ethos to its curriculum development and delivery?

Maximising your own employability potential

As a result of the discussion over employability within higher education, a concept of a graduate identity approach has arisen (Holmes, 2001) that is owned by the graduate (Hinchliffe and Jolly, 2011). It is suggested that it is made up of the four strands of development previously discussed: values, intellect, performance and engagement. Graduate identity and potential are maximised by graduates providing evidence of engagement in a wide range of activities, experiences and organisations. The generation of evidence to maximise graduate identity will enable employers to judge the ability for a particular graduate to fulfil and develop within the requirements of the work situation with greater confidence. This concept is encouraging individuals to demonstrate what they can offer based on evidence to date. The importance of evidencing employability is critical in order to be able to demonstrate to employers not what you have done in the past but what your future potential may be (Holmes, 2001; Hinchliffe and Jolly, 2011). The process of gaining employment involves a process of judgement on the behalf of the employer – it is not purely a process of measuring a person and matching them to a job (Holmes, 2006). On occasions it may be possible that employers lack clarity about exactly who or what they want and are also making a judgement of the future potential of individuals too. Being able to evidence who you are and what you can bring to a job situation with confidence and enthusiasm is critical for your success.

There should be a partnership between the skills and attributes approach to employability and a graduate identity approach, and should consider at the time of graduation how a graduate will articulate their employability and potential in order to gain employment as a graduate (Holmes, 2001, 2006). This reinforces the argument presented in this chapter that consideration of employability needs to start at the beginning of your student experience to provide a focus on employability throughout your studies. Embedding employability will enable you to genuinely evidence and confidently articulate your employability at the point of graduation and beyond. This argument relates to individuals at any point of their employability journey – not just at the point of graduation.

> **Time for reflection**
> How can you best demonstrate the potential that you have got to employers?
> What have you got to bring to that job situation?

The key message from both the graduate identity approach and the psychosocial construct of employability is an awareness of the world of work and employer expectations, as explored further in Chapter 2. Without an understanding of what is required, there may be a resulting disconnect between your employability and the employability required by the employing organisation.

What do employers want from graduates?

It is important for higher education institutions to be aware of what employers want from graduates in relation to employability (Wilson, 2012) to ensure a partnership between the two. Engagement between higher education institutions and employers has been well established in the past, with a suggestion that the gap between education and employers is widening over recent years (Rosenburg, Heimler and Morote, 2012).

It has been suggested that employers can have a narrow interest and understanding of employability (McQuaid and Lindsay, 2005). However, from previous discussions in this chapter, the same could be said about higher education institutions! There needs to be a common language of employability between academia and employers. This can be very difficult to achieve (Harvey, 2001). It is, therefore, difficult to answer the question of what employers want from graduates. Sometimes employers may not be entirely sure themselves, and may be under constant change resulting in limited evidence to provide direction to graduates. Despite this backdrop, it is still important to try to establish what is important in order to focus on key areas of development (Holmes, 2006), as employers are not just looking for a subject-specific achievement (Yorke, 2006). Also, with a changing health and social care work landscape, graduates may need to initially work in roles that are not considered to be graduate level (Moreau and Leathwood, 2006) or relating to their degree subject, thereby increasing further the importance of an individual's wider employability, rather than just their degree. It is likely that some skills will be prioritised within certain areas of work (Wilson, 2012). To a certain extent the responsibility lies with you to establish which skills are prioritised within certain areas of work, by exploring the organisational culture and values and personal specifications of similar roles via relevant web sites. Students generally are not ignorant of employer's requirements but still give employability a low priority over other things in their lives (Atkins, 1999). It is difficult when you have the demands of studying to think beyond just getting from one assignment to another as well as how you need to be developing your employability – but you should aim to do this when at all possible, as you will reap the benefits when it comes to applying for jobs at the end of your studies.

Time for reflection

What priority do you give employability within your everyday life? What aspects of your personality do you think would appeal to employers and why?

Rosenberg, Heimler and Morote (2012) undertook a research study to establish what were perceived as important employability skills that are required for employment. Three groups were studied: recent graduates, the faculty that taught them and human resources managers that recruited them. The three groups articulated differences in opinion in relation to required elements of employability. However, all three groups agreed that leadership was a critical skill. Numeracy and literacy were identified as skills that are a basic requirement. In another paper, personality has been as identified as one of the most important criteria for employers (Moreau and Leathwood, 2006). Values and ethics, including work ethic, have also been highlighted as important aspects of employability (Rosenberg, Heimler and Morote, 2012: Hinchliffe and Jolly, 2011); it is not just down to skill performance, it is about who you are and what you can contribute to an organisation. The requirement of common generic employability skills within jobs has little published evidence to inform individuals (Atkins, 1999). If you are thinking about areas such as values, engagement, intellect and performance, you will be ensuring that you are focusing on doing employability-related activities/experiences, which is key evidence for your employability and potential (Hinchliffe and Jolly, 2011). Employability needs to be systematically approached to enable employers to see how your learning has been developed and built upon. There is an assumption that learning can be transferred from one situation to another, but you need to ensure that this is explicitly evidenced and confidently communicated to employers (Yorke, 2006, Holmes, 2011). Unprepared students are unlikely to be successful in getting jobs (Rosenberg *et al.*, 2012).

Time for reflection

What long term employability goals do you want to focus on and why? For example, do you want to develop yourself to be a team leader, do you want to have the ability to set up your own social enterprise?

You need to be able to hit the ground running (Harvey, 2000) within a changing work landscape. You need to have a range of strong core employability skills to be able to respond to the job-specific specialist skills, which may be changing (Rosenberg *et al.*, 2012). Flexibility and response to change are required from employers, and an ability for you to sometimes grow your own jobs within an organisation will be required from you, as you will be part of organisational change (Harvey, 2000). For example, a junior Occupational Therapist had a desire to work towards becoming a palliative care specialist. A palliative care specialist Occupational Therapy post did not currently exist within the hospital where she was working. However, when the opportunity arose to develop her knowledge and skills within the area of palliative care, she took them. Any relevant courses on palliative care – she attended. Any networks related to palliative care – she joined and built up contacts. Any research related to palliative care – she participated in. She undertook audits to demonstrate the need for a specialist Occupational Therapist in palliative care. Within two years she had secured funding for a senior position as an Occupational Therapist working within palliative care, and within five years was a specialist palliative care Occupational Therapist. Her passion, drive and proactiveness were what led to her success. Within the changing world of work, resilience is an essential trait for individuals to demonstrate (Rothwell and Arnold, 2007) – employers want to have confidence that you will survive in the world of work. Health and social care professions are tough – there are constant changes and pressures, and resilience to manage and respond positively to the changes and pressures are key for your well-being and progression through your career.

Employability is a life-long issue (Dacre Pool and Sewell, 2007) and does not finish when you have been successful in gaining employment. Employability needs to continue throughout your career – those individuals with high employability are influential within organisations (Nauta *et al.*, 2009) and can, therefore, maximise their career potential. For you to continue to maximise your career potential, a continuing drive to develop yourself and take opportunities within your new work situation is crucial.

Healthcare employability

In this chapter, the focus to date has been more on generic employability issues. Within health care, the situation in relation to employability is not dissimilar to non-health related employability. Within the United Kingdom, there are system changes to health and social care that are having an influence on employability requirements of healthcare students, with changes to the employment options that are available for graduates. Regardless of where individuals work within health care in the world, there are changes to adapt to, with a resulting change in the employability requirements to prepare yourself for the future landscape of work.

Within each of the healthcare professions, the relevant professional and governing bodies publish basic minimum levels of professional and clinical competence. All students on a pre-registration healthcare course need to fulfil these criteria in order to graduate. From an employability point of view, this means that there are a large number of students who will be graduating with a similar professional and clinical competence profile. It is, therefore, crucial for healthcare students to focus on acquiring additional elements of employability during their studies, in order to strengthen their position within a competitive job market.

Papers within the United Kingdom – but which are equally relevant worldwide – have been written to provide an employability profile for healthcare students to refer to (Kubler and Forbes, 2005a, 2005b, 2005c). The main generic competencies identified by employers were outlined as:

- Cognitive skills
- Generic competencies
- Personal capabilities
- Technical ability
- Business and/or organisational awareness
- Practical and professional elements.

Within each of the generic competencies are listed numerous benchmarks and there are suggestions as to how these could be achieved. The documents are very long and predominantly focused on clinical and professional issues, but they are useful as documents to refer to when looking at employability within health care. Research undertaken by Taylor (2014) aimed to provide information on healthcare employability by undertaking focus group discussions and using a questionnaire survey with students, educators and employers as participants. There were common themes between the groups as to what was meant by employability and what is expected of healthcare graduates, over and above the requirements for professional registration. The participants were asked to rate the themes in order of importance. The three themes that were rated highest were: making a good impression, enthusiasm for the job and passion for the profession. The least important rated theme was academic grades. This does not mean that academic grades are not important, but in relation to the other employability themes it was rated as less important than all of the other themes.

The themes generated by the research by Taylor (2014) support the considerations of employability that have been presented in previous literature and provide employability considerations not just focusing on skills or attributes but on a holistic approach to employability. The degree and associated clinical competence and skills that come with it are important but what are rated as equally important are interpersonal elements. It is easy to demonstrate the achievement of your degree, as you will receive a certificate, but it is important to consider how you are going to demonstrate fulfilment of all of the other aspects of employability that have been highlighted as important.

Time for reflection
How do you currently rate yourself on the employability themes outlined? Could you provide evidence to demonstrate your employability within each of the themes presented?

Evidencing your employability

This chapter has outlined the concept of employability and described a number of models of employability. The underlying message throughout has been the ability of individuals to evidence their employability. Professional development portfolios enable individuals to report the employability journey that they have had (Hinchliffe and Jolly, 2011). There is a strong link between employability and professional development portfolios (Dacre Pool and Sewell, 2007). The process of producing a professional development portfolio will provide an individual with opportunities to reflect – which is an expectation in graduates (Atkins, 1999) – and then to generate an action plan to evidence a response to learning which is necessary (Yorke, 2006). Continuing professional development portfolios are good to demonstrate how individuals make sense of their experiences rather than just a list of the experiences (Fugate, Kinicki and Ashforth, 2004). Listing experiences does not demonstrate how the individual has learned and moved on from the experience – employers need to have confidence that individuals are able to do. Within healthcare education, reflection and continuing professional development are encouraged and supported from day one and you should then continue this throughout your working life. Being in the habit of reflecting and generating evidence of your continuing development is not only good for evidencing your employability but is also an essential requirement for most healthcare professional registration bodies.

Time for reflection
How will you systematically address and record your employability development?

Taylor (2014) used the focus group research to develop an evidence based UEA Healthcare Employability Development Portfolio. This portfolio provides healthcare students and educators with a software framework of employability based on the themes generated from the research (known as employability domains). Each employability domain has three incremental phases of development, so that students can develop their employability over a period of time (for example phase 1 for year 1, phase 2 for year 2 and phase 3 for year 3 of a 3-year pre-registration healthcare course). Supportive resources are provided at each phase of development to encourage reflection and action planning from the individual. This ensures that employability development is focused on throughout studies and also provides a structured approach to employability. Individuals completing the employability development portfolio generate evidence to document and this facilitates their confidence to articulate their employability journey at the point of applying for a job.

As previously suggested, continuing professional development is required within the healthcare working environment (Moore *et al.*, 2011). Developing a positive and structured approach to professional development as a student will prepare you well for continuing this focus and discipline within the working environment. Employability is a life-long issue (Dacre Pool and Sewell 2007) and there needs to be a continuing focus on personal development and employability, which can help you in your career pathway – as discussed in Chapter 2. In order to develop a career, it is essential for you to go through the process of personal development planning to identify your areas of strength and development (Watts, 2006) that can be worked upon in a structured way.

Time for reflection
What key areas of employability do you need to focus on?

Conclusions

Employability is difficult to define and has been the topic of debate over a number of years. There are a number of models of employability. Many focus purely on the skill acquisition side of employability. However, a holistic approach to employability is recommended. Personal values and ethics emerge as a priority area of employability. Employability assumes a high priority within higher education institutions, but the implementation of employability within the curriculum and development of student employability is not entirely clear from the literature available, with only a few institutions fully embedding employability explicitly in the curriculum. Guidance for students and educators in the development of employability within education is limited. The understanding of employability for employers is not extensively documented but there has been a shift in recent years to the need for you to be flexible and resilient within changing working landscapes. The concept of an internal locus of control supports a proactive and opportunistic approach from you to the working environment to give yourself the best chance of maximising employability.

There needs to be more engagement between employers and higher education institutions to establish a common language of employability, which, in turn, will provide clarity for all of those involved in graduate employability. Healthcare students will all graduate with clinical and professional competence. Therefore, you need to focus on the other elements of employability to maximise your chances within a competitive work marketplace. Employers want to see evidence of employability to demonstrate the potential that you have and what you can bring to the workplace. Portfolios are encouraged as a way of organising a structured approach to employability development and encourage reflection and action planning as a result of learning. This provides you with evidence of your development and a continuing focus on personal development in relation to employability – employability is the journey, employment is the destination. In the ever changing world of work there will be multiple destinations with many employability journeys in between. Engagement in employability is essential from an early stage to maximise your own employability and career development opportunities.

Definitions

Employability   Within this book the term employability is used in the context of healthcare students who have just graduated or are about to graduate. The term is used to mean the knowledge, skills, attributes, experiences that you have had to date within your curriculum and extracurricular activities that will maximise your development and culminate in the ability to articulate yourself as an employable individual with confidence when applying for jobs. Employability continues when you are in employment, to demonstrate your continuing personal and professional development to maximise your potential for career progression.

Employment   This term is used in this book to describe when you have acquired a job and are in employment.

Employability is the process of working towards being at the stage to apply for a job and *employment* is the outcome.

Potential interview questions in this area
- How do your personal elements of employability relate to the personal specification for a specific job?
- Do you think that skills or attributes are more important for this role?
- How do you think that you should develop your employability whilst in employment?
- What do you think you could contribute to our organisation?
- Can you give me some examples of transferable skills that you can bring into the work environment?
- What are your opinions on reflection?

References

Andrews J and Higson H (2007) *Education, employment and graduate employability: Project manual*. Aston University, Birmingham.

Atkins M (1999) Oven-ready and self-basting: taking stock of employability skills. *Teaching in Higher Education*, **4**(2):267–280.

Bennett N, Dunne E and Carré C (1999) Patterns of core and generic skill provision in higher education. *Higher Education*, **37**:71–93.

Dacre Pool L and Sewell P (2007) The key to employability: developing a practical model of graduate employability. *Education and Training*, **49**(4):277–289.

Day H (2009) *Ceth employability framework*. http://escalate.ac.uk/downloads/6465. pdf; last accessed 18 August 2015.

Fugate M, Kinicki A and Ashforth B (2004) Employability: A psycho-social construct, its dimensions, and applications. *Journal of Vocational Behaviour*, **65**:14–38.

Graves S (2011) Exploring employability: educational resources. *Journal of Hospitality, Leisure, Sport and Tourism Education*, **10**(1):129–131.

Harvey L (2000) New realities: the relationship between higher education and employment. *Tertiary Education and Management*, **6**:3–17.

Harvey L (2001) Defining and measuring employability. *Quality in Higher Education*, **7**(2):97–109.

Harvey L and Knight P (2003) *Briefings on employability 5 – helping departments to develop employability*. Enhancing Student Employability Co-ordination Team, Higher Education Academy, York, UK.

Higher Education Academy (2012) *Report on teaching and learning summit 16–17 May 2012*. Higher Education Academy, York, UK.

Hillage J and Pollard E (1998) *Employability: Developing a framework for policy analysis*. Research Report RR85, UK Department of Education and Employment.

Hinchliffe G and Jolly A (2011) Graduate identity and employability. *British Educational Research Journal*, **37**(4):563–584.

Holmes L (2001) Reconsidering graduate employability: the 'graduate identity' approach. *Quality in Higher Education*, **7**(2):111–119.

Holmes L (2006) *Reconsidering graduate employability: beyond possessive-instrumentalism.* Paper presented at the Seventh International Conference on HRD research and practice across Europe, 22–24 May 2006, University of Tilburg, The Netherlands.

Kubler B and Forbes P (2005a) *Student employability profile: Health Sciences.* Enhancing Student Employability Co-ordination Team, Higher Education Academy, York, UK.

Kubler B and Forbes P (2005b) *Employability guide health science and practice: Allied health professions student employability profile.* Enhancing Student Employability Co-ordination Team, Higher Education Academy, York, UK.

Kubler B and Forbes P (2005c) *Employability guide health science and practice: Nursing student employability profile.* Enhancing student Employability Co-ordination Team, Higher Education Academy, York, UK.

Maher A (2011) Employability statements: A review for HEFCE by the Higher Education Academy of the submissions to the Unistats website. *Journal of Hospitality, Leisure, Sport and Tourism Education,* **10**(1):132–133.

Moore J, Brown S, Chapman H *et al.* (2011) *Education and training.* NHS Future Forum. https://www.gov.uk/government/uploads/system/uploads/attachment_data/file/213751/dh_127543.pdf; last accessed 18 August 2015.

Moreau M and Leathwood C (2006) Graduates' employability and the discourse of employability: a critical analysis. *Journal of Education and Work,* **19**(4):305–324.

McQuaid R and Lindsay C (2005) The concept of employability. *Urban Studies,* **42**(2):197–219.

Nauta A, Van Vianen A, Van der Heijden B, Van Dam K and Willemsen M (2009) Understanding the factors that promote employability orientation: The impact of employability culture, career satisfaction, and role breadth self-efficacy. *Journal of Occupational and Organizational Psychology,* **82**:233–251.

Pegg A, Waldock J, Hendy-Isaac S and Lawton R (2012) *Pedagogy for employability.* The Higher Education Academy, York, UK.

Rosenberg S, Heimler R and Morote E (2012), Basic employability skills: a triangular design approach. *Education and Training,* **54**(1):7–20.

Rothwell A and Arnold J (2007) Self-perceived employability: development and validation of a scale. *Personnel Review,* **36**(1):23–41.

Smith J, McKnight A and Naylor R (2000) Graduate employability: policy and performance in higher education in the UK. *The Economic Journal,* **110**(464):F382–F411.

Taylor L (2014) The formulation of the healthcare employability development portfolio: An evidence-based model of employability for healthcare students to use throughout their studies to maximize their employability. 25th International Networking for Healthcare Education Conference, 2–4 September, Cambridge, UK (http://www.jillrogersassociates.co.uk/net2014abstractsandcorepapers.html; last accessed 18 August 2015).

Watts AG (2006) *Career Development Learning and Employability.* The Higher Education Academy, York, UK.

Wilson T (2012) *A review of business-university collaboration.* UK Department for Business, Innovation and Skills, London.

Yorke M and Knight P (2006) *Learning and employability – Embedding employability in the curriculum.* Higher Education Academy, York, UK.

Yorke M (2006) *Learning and employability – Employability in higher education: what is it – what is it not.* Higher Education Academy, York, UK.

Chapter 2 **Career planning and management**

Adrienne Jolly
Career Service, University of East Anglia, Norwich, UK

Introduction – Aims of this chapter

In the previous chapter, we examined some definitions of the concept of employability, which, in the words of Mantz Yorke (2004), consists of *'a set of achievements – skills, understandings and personal attributes – that make graduates more likely to gain employment and be successful in their chosen occupations, hence benefitting themselves, the workforce, the community and the economy'.* Already we can see that the idea of employability is a complex one, embracing many preoccupations that include an individual's values and personal motivations. We will now consider the similarly complex idea of 'career': What is meant by it (both in general and in the context of the health-care professional)? We will suggest some of the external influences that can affect your own choices (some of which we have already explored in Chapter 1) and also put forward some tools with which to examine your idea of a career.

We will also examine common perspectives that can help early career professionals to understand and better manage their career, considering some of the key factors that influence career choices, and pointing out ways in which harnessing self-awareness can help you to make the right decisions. Throughout the chapter 'practitioner's perspective' will be offered, drawing examples from my experience in careers guidance.

For some people, a career is often seen in hindsight, particularly when a break or change has required them to reflect on where they want to go next: 'How did I get here and what do I do now?' That you are reading this book suggests that this is not the case for you, because you are probably looking ahead with a view to understanding where your career might now take you within your chosen health profession.

How to Develop Your Healthcare Career: A Guide to Employability and Professional Development, First Edition. Edited by Lisa Taylor.

How people manage their careers has been the subject of countless publications, web sites and blogs, and there are numerous models and guides on the market that can help you to explore this area further.

> ### The importance of reflection
> Being accustomed to asking questions about your career can be extremely beneficial. As a health professional, you probably have a distinct advantage over many of your peers, because you have been required to think about your professional development and practice throughout your training and pre-registration placements. By keeping a placement diary, you will have been asking questions about that experience which, whilst primarily intended to help you through your training, will also have contributed to the creation of a comprehensive picture of your career. Where have you thrived? What learning has really stimulated and motivated you? Where were you less happy and why do you think that was? Are you influenced by the people around you more than the tasks you undertake? And what has your experience so far told you about the structure of the healthcare professions and of organisations in general.

What do we mean by 'Career'?

At its most straightforward, a career is an occupation undertaken for significant length of time during a person's life and with opportunities for progress. However, it is clear that the concept of a career means different things to different people, and is important for both the individual and wider society and economy. Fifty years ago, a career typically meant employment in one type of role or for one employer over the majority of one's working life. Progress was linear and incremental, and retirement at 60 or 65 meant the end of your working life. What 'career' means today, and indeed will mean in the future, is far more fluid. Changes in the employment market, education, the application of technology, working practices and organisational structures are just a few of the factors changing the shape of careers. Recognising that your career does not exist in a vacuum, but is influenced by a range of external factors is particularly important in the health professions, and many of these are explored in later chapters.

Describing careers

Many different theoretical and practical approaches to careers have emerged over the course of the last century to explain why we do what we do and what influences us in that choice. A lot of this theory focuses on the individual, asking what they are good at, and finding ways to match these skills to the labour market. Indeed the first publication on the subject of careers, *Choosing a Vocation*, which was published by Frank Parsons in 1909 (in the United States), advocates choosing a career based on a person's 'aptitudes, abilities, ambitions, resources and limitations'. This approach, which has since become known as 'Vocational Personality Theory' (Holland, 1997), is still commonplace today and is often the starting point in conversations about career. You have probably been asked (perhaps by helpful relatives), 'So, what do you enjoy doing?', and this is then followed by a suggestion that 'matches you' to a career: 'Have you thought about....?' Quite often we align ourselves to vocations in this way without much consideration, 'I've always enjoyed helping people so nursing seemed an obvious choice'. Sometimes such self-awareness can be accurate and effective, hence the increasing use of psychometric testing as an aid to recruitment.

However, there are many critics of this approach. Sociological career theorists are one such an example. They have sought to challenge trait and factor matching, arguing that the external influences of class, gender, race, and the employment market itself have a greater influence on career for many, and suggesting that to truly match capabilities to opportunities would require the removal of all such obstacles. Career, therefore, is better explained as something that is constructed by society and, as such, may include an inherent (or inherited?) advantage or disadvantage. These theorists also argue that we inherit ideas about career that mirror our class or social experience. The British theorist Phil Hodkinson termed these 'horizons for action' (Hodkinson, 2009), effectively meaning that the choices you make are directly influenced by what you experience around you: quite literally, what careers are visible to you through your life experience and community. Whilst this might seem irrelevant if you have already chosen and are embarking on your new career, it is worth thinking about the people and experiences that you have encountered and will encounter which might 'widen' your own career horizons.

A third common strand of career development theory is one of narrative. Here, career takes the form of story – we tell stories about ourselves to help understand our motivations and actions, past and present experiences, and the connections (obvious or less so) between our many decisions. These more 'psychology-driven' ideas place the emphasis on the individual and how they may have been influenced and shaped by experience. We are characters in our own story. Here, an individual's career is seen as being something shaped and defined by their image of themselves and what they believe others think of them. An example of narrative career might be the researcher who decides to pursue a career in science because their sibling suffered from a childhood disease; or someone who does not consider management roles because they cannot 'see' themselves in such a position. Narrative or psychological theories can be helpful when considering how confident we feel about our 'vocational identity' – that person who we can visualise working in the outside world, and whose image may be seen reflected in the eyes of family, friends, teachers and contemporaries.

A fourth and very interesting approach is the work of Donal Super, which spanned from 1953 to 1996, beginning with his influential *Theory of Career Development* (Super, 1953) and subsequent work with Mark Savickas (Super, Savickas and Super, 1996) in developing this still further. Super has been a major influence on career development theories and, in this context, it is useful to draw attention to his idea that our working lives consist of both roles *and* timescales. Super means by this that we have a chronological aspect to our career (literally starting with our education and ending with our retirement from the labour market), but that we also inhabit different roles throughout our lifetime, one of which is our career (Super, 1984). However, as children, carers, parents, friends, partners, colleagues and members of a community, there are many other factors that impact on our careers. At different stages in our lives we encounter different challenges and opportunities. A simple example is the idea that having and raising children will affect your career choices and priorities. In this case, the role of parent may become more dominant ('salient') and cause us to reassess our work-role priorities.

A second strand of Super's work (and one which we will come back to later in this chapter) is the idea of a career as cyclical. Super argues that our careers are made up of a series of smaller cycles (from deciding upon and engaging in a role through to disengaging and moving on) and this recognition that career is a lifelong process, one that requires you to be ready for and respond to change and opportunity, is resonant with some of the fundamental ideas of employability discussed in the previous chapter (Super, 1994). Where Super's ideas are particularly helpful are in his call to action (if you want to make good decisions you need to understand the process of your decision making), and in that he is an example of a career theorist whose work developed over many years, taking account of external/societal and internal/psychological factors. As we shall see, his work continues to have a huge influence on the idea of 'career' today.

Using multiple perspectives

It is, however, important to remember that the ideas briefly introduced to you here are just a few of the theoretical approaches that have been developed in explaining and exploring careers: this is by no means an exhaustive list, and nor have those ideas listed been explored in any more than a brief summary.

In understanding what is influencing our career ideas, adhering to one particular career theory or model can sometimes feel restrictive. Instead, it can help to take a range of perspectives, acknowledging that one's career choices will be influenced in many ways, and working with this awareness to maximise the opportunities open to you.

The four approaches outlined above are summarised in Box 2.1, in which questions that you might use to interrogate your own career decisions to date are also suggested.

Box 2.1 Interrogating your career decisions

Career as 'matching'
Career is a process of identifying skills, interests, preferences or personality type, and aligning these with occupations that require/attract similar people. From this matching approach, psychometric testing and career-match questionnaires were developed. Career decisions are made based on finding the right match of individual and vocation.

May sound like
'I always knew I wanted to work in a job that used my people skills, and so set about looking at degrees that would lead me in that direction'.
Or:
'I love the clinical side of my job, but I find the managerial tasks really stressful; I just don't feel comfortable delegating to others'.

Questions
• What do I love doing?
• What did I enjoy best when younger (and am I still doing something similar)?
• What do I find hard (and what comes easily to me)?
• Are there environments that I particularly enjoy working in? (Customer focused, autonomous etc.)

Career as a 'cycle'
Career is a cyclical process of exploring ideas, gaining confidence and identity in a role, and maintaining that role until circumstance or personal motivation require you to change. 'Good' career decision making is based on ensuring the exploration stage of a decision is properly thought through.

May sound like
'I had been interested in Occupational Therapy for a long time, but I was encouraged to do work experience and talk to people before I applied. This experience confirmed to me that I had made the right choice and my research really validated that for me.'
Or:
'I keep finding myself in roles that just don't feel comfortable. I stay for about a year, feel frustrated, and move on. I thought that this was the industry for me, but I just can't seem to get it right.'

Questions
• How did I choose what career to follow? What research did I do before applying to train?
• Did I explore other options and choose this one? If not, why was that?
• How do I make decisions?

Career 'externally influenced'

Career opportunity is influenced by economic and social factors, education, cultural or religious factors, as well as geography, national/political policy etc. (access to the workplace). Certain careers may appear less accessible because of gender/race/[dis]ability, or access to funding, whilst others are considered 'normal' for a particular societal group or community.

May sound like

'My school had really strong links with the local college and they came in to run sessions with us in year 11. I think that encouraged me to take the course I did, and I was the first in our family to do anything like that'.

Or:

'I was really interested in physics and chemistry, but I didn't really feel encouraged at school to take them to a higher level. Most of the girls in our school, if we took a science at all, took biology'.

Questions

- Who were the people around me when I was growing up?
- What career role models were there for me?
- Were there barriers (social, economic, religious) that I think I had to overcome to do what I'm doing now?
- Does my interest in this career stem from/is affected by my background?

Career as a 'Story'

Careers or skills develop through experience, and ideas about what is possible evolve through the influence of people around you (or other role models such as people in the media or literature).

Career forms part of a wider narrative (helping to define the individual) and 'success' is influenced by how the individual perceives themselves in a particular role, organisation or setting.

May sound like

'My brother has a learning difficulty. Helping him at home, and helping my parents too – I think it had a huge influence on me and my decision to go into Speech Therapy'.

Or:

'At school I was told that I'd be better working in something manual: that I'd struggle if I trained in something too technical'.

Questions

- Who did/do I admire?
- Do I have 'heroes' (or villains)?
- Did I consider this career because of a particular experience or set of experiences?
- How does this role make me feel about myself? Do I feel the need to feel fulfilled from my work?

What shape is your career?

This might seem like an odd question to ask – but we often see careers represented by ladders, or an arrow on a graph moving diagonally up and across the page. Thinking of your career in this way can be challenging. In guidance, we often encounter young graduates and final-year students who are really frightened of taking the first step in starting their career: 'What if I choose the wrong specialism?' 'What if I start in the wrong job?' 'What if I limit my chances by staying close to home?'

Thinking of your career in a linear or laddered way can exacerbate such fears. Clearly, if your career was a straight trajectory, beginning at 21 and not stopping until retirement, then where you start *would* be critical: but career is not that shape at all. Given all we know about the influencing factors, then your career at its most simple is going to look far more like a staircase, but one that has many plateaus or landings, and it may be that you will take a few steps down at points in your life before climbing another flight.

Factors that influence our career

There are many factors affecting what we do, and this section tries to briefly summarise some of the more commonplace that might affect your own choices.

As you read through this list, consider the following questions:

- What factors have influenced you in the past?
- What factors are influencing you at present?
- What are the factors that might have a bearing on the future?
- Are there actions that you need to take or be prepared for?

Personal factors: *Things about you that might affect your choices and opportunities*
Motivations and values: **What is important to you?**

Beginning with such a broad question might feel overwhelming, but what is important to you influences your day-to-day decisions, your longer term choices, and will not remain static as you move through life. Your values can influence what you do, why you do it, who you do it with and for, and how much you expect to get paid for it! Using value audits can be a really helpful way to test your motivations (an exercise is included at the end of the book), but they can also help you to understand why you feel more confident in one role or organisation than another.

The importance of values

It is sometimes easy to overlook the importance of values when we consider career. Quite often when a client presents in careers guidance feeling very confused about their career choice and unsure how to move forward, it turns out that there is friction between what motivates the client and where they have found themselves in their career. For example, if someone is motivated by the need to work collaboratively and for a common purpose, but finds themselves in an organisation that is working competitively for tenders, then this may lead to them feeling unhappy or uncomfortable. In such circumstances, they may choose to focus their energy on trying to find a new employer – but sometimes this is not practical, and at such times, it is often good simply to acknowledge where there are incompatibilities, and consider strategies that might help. It is probably not realistic to think that all of our values will 'find a home' in our career – but the closer you align your values to what you do, the greater your sense of career fulfilment.

Values matter to employers, too. A common shorthand for what employers look for is 'Can you, will you, fit':

• **'Can you'** – do you have the skills for the job and the ability to learn and develop.

• **'Will you'** – do you have the attitude and approach to the work that is going to motivate you

• **'Fit'** – do you understand what the organisation does and needs, and will you fit with this?

Clearly values are especially relevant to health professionals and contribute to ideas of professionalism and of professional standards, as explored in Chapter 3.

Attributes and strengths: **What comes easily to you and what behaviours do you enjoy bringing to your work?**
Attributes and strengths offer a slightly different perspective but can be just as valuable in assessing your career choices. The exercises in Chapter 9 ask you to consider what qualities you bring to your work: what attributes come naturally to you? Attributes may influence your career because they can affect how *comfortable* you feel in a role, for example: If you see yourself as an organiser or galvaniser, then you may naturally find yourself taking these roles in the workplace, and perhaps be the one who suggests new ways of doing things; If you do not feel comfortable organising people, then a role that expects that of you will likely be stressful. Recognising the relationships between what you do and how you do it will help you.

Time for reflection
If you were asked the question 'What is your greatest strength?', what answer would you give?

Skill development: **What you are good at and where you are happy learning?**

We talk often about skills in the context of 'employability' as well as career, and commonly use phrases such as 'transferable skills' or 'soft skills' in our workplace. Whilst the idea of acquiring skills seems very straightforward, keeping your skills up to date can be difficult and developing new skills in order to progress (to a higher band, or into a new organisation or role) can feel like a challenge. Even the idea that skills are 'transferrable' can be a complicated one: how can you transfer the experience of essay writing to completing a report for a line manager? How are these things the same? In career guidance, I encourage clients to think of their skills as something that you translate rather than transfer, meaning that the skills that you have learned may have to change in some way in order to be applied to a new context.

Where skills are clearly important in career development is simply:
* *Do you have the skills needed for a role?*
* *Are the skills required to function in the role changing?*
* *Are you developing new skills that help you to progress as you would like?*

Time for reflection
To what extent has your professional training helped you to ask questions like this?

In order to develop in your career, you will also need to articulate your skills: no employer can or will shortlist you for a role if you have not met the personal selection criteria and cannot give examples to evidence this (see Chapter 8, where we will consider applications in more detail).

Vocational factors: *What might affect how and where you work?*

The vocational 'sweet spot' could perhaps best be described as knowing what you love, being good at it, and then matching these with what society has decided it needs and is prepared to pay for. In this middle space there still exist questions to consider: Do the roles that you are interested in exist where you want to live? Are there changes in the structure or nature of your job that you must address? Do you want to work for a particular kind of organisation because of its values or mission, and is that a valid option for you at this stage in your career? Vocational factors can also be very personal; for example: Can you find the flexible hours you need when the time comes to start a family?

> **Time for reflection**
> Are there vocational factors that are influencing your decision making at this stage in your life?

External or market factors: *What might affect the opportunities open to you?*

Understanding how the organisations or occupations that interest you are placed in the health and social care sector, and how organisational change can (and will) impact your career are important final factors to consider.

The health professions in the United Kingdom have undergone radical and irreversible change in recent decades, with new technology and treatments changing how we work day to day, and new structures changing who is providing treatment and care within which structures. Maintaining an awareness, not just of what is happening in your department but also of where your department sits in the wider hospital or service, will be critical to your career development in the future, wherever in the world you are. Continuing professional development requires you to keep abreast of how your own professional skill base develops. However, maintaining an engaged interest in this wider context will not only alert you to changes but also show your employers that you are aware of the 'bigger picture'. Change can also be emotionally difficult and professionally challenging. Whilst an employment contract does not come with its own crystal ball, keeping aware and informed of these external factors can help you to recognise oncoming change and perhaps address any specific vocational or personal factors in preparation.

> **Time for reflection**
> What are there external factors that you think are likely to affect your career in the future?

Mapping factors

These factors have been summarised in Figure 2.1 and some of the key questions that relate to these factors set out.

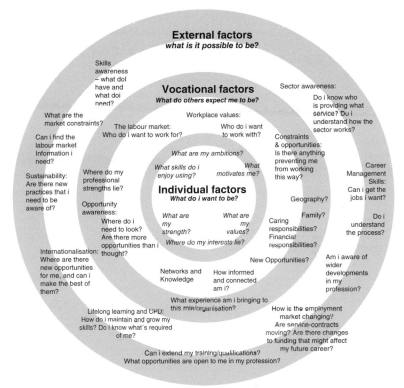

Figure 2.1 Factors influencing our careers

Time for reflection

Consider the questions in Figure 2.1. To what extent can you answer them at this stage?

Are there questions in a particular zone that you find harder to answer? Why do you think that might be? Do you think that these are important questions to find answers to?

Making good career decisions

In this chapter so far we have looked at what influences our career decisions and suggested some ways to explain and understand where you might find yourself at present. In this final part of the chapter, I want to consider how you might make best use of planning to make good career decisions, using some of these tools and questions.

Returning to the career development theorist, Donald Super, Super suggested that in order to make good career decisions you must complete a process or cycle, and that we are required to go through this cycle many times throughout our lives (Super, 1955, 1984).

This cycle consists of four stages: exploration, establishment, maintenance and disengagement. These are outlined here and examples offered in the boxes of how this process might unfold.

Exploration

This stage involves exploring and testing ideas, specifying what or where you want to be and taking the appropriate steps to succeed in this. Exploration means taking the time to consider personal and vocational factors to understand where your next step is (Box 2.2).

Establishment

This involves acquiring the skills needed to develop in order to gain vocational self-efficacy in a role. For example, applying the skills and knowledge that you bring into a role and adding the relevant organisational and vocational knowledge to allow you to perform the role well (Box 2.3).

Maintenance

This is the point at which you are able to perform in a role and where stability in this career or role is the primary objective. This may mean focusing on financial stability, improving your status in the workplace and continuing to

---

Box 2.2 Sam

Sam has completed all of his placements and is nearing the end of his degree. He was keen to work with children and initially chose physiotherapy with a vague idea that he might want to be based in a community setting (his mother works as a practice nurse in a large surgery). However, through his placement experience, Sam has realised that he has a real interest in rehabilitation and has also thought about how he might progress in his career in the longer term. He now needs to think carefully about his next steps. To explore this further, Sam might wish to:

• Using his reflective journal, think about why he found this particular placement stimulating.
• List or map the values and motivations that he would like to maintain in his career.
• Revisit the web site for his professional body and research in more detail the pathways open to him.
• Compare job descriptions for different roles – what appeals?
• Talk to peers, teaching staff and clinical staff through his placements to test some of his ideas.
• Speak to a careers advisor at his university.

Box 2.3 David

David has entered his first post-qualifying role. This was one of a dozen roles he applied for, and he is now working a charitable organisation that works with young people. This is ideal for David at the moment, as this is the client group that really appeals to him. However, for David, the challenge has been getting to grips with the working practices and processes of the charity. His placements were all in hospitals and council-run units and, up until applying for permanent roles, he did not really give much thought to what it would be like working for a small autonomous organisation. He really enjoys the environment, but feels as if there is less supervision and support than he might have expected (and indeed have experienced) in the NHS. He has had to learn about other organisations in the area and get a better understanding of how they all relate to NHS and council provision. It hass also meant that he is having to work with more external organisations than he imagined, and this means gaining confidence in presentations, talking at meetings and managing his time. David is thriving in this role, but he makes sure that he and his supervisor meet regularly, and that he uses the reflective skills he developed in his training. This way, he feels confident that he is applying his skills and developing in the role in a way that works for him.

Box 2.4 Jyoti

Jyoti has been in her current role for five years. She has reached a senior grade and feels that she has contractual and professional stability at the moment. She is leading a team and enjoys the management responsibilities that this offers but her clinical work is equally as important. She has no need to earn more money at this stage although it might give her more options in the future. There may soon be an opportunity to apply for a higher grade coming up, but this effectively would mean making the transition from practitioner to manager. The challenge appeals to her. As she considers this opportunity, she may want to:
- Consider those aspects of her work that reflect her core values and motivators: What would this promotion mean in terms of changing their focus? Does this feel comfortable?
- Can she have informal discussions with people who have made that leap?
- Will this opportunity arise again? Is there a way back?
- What will change? Would a role audit help? Could she compare her current role with an example of a new role and make a point-by-point comparison?
- Where does she see herself in five years' time? When she imagines herself in the same role, how does that make her feel?

develop in the role. For some, maintenance is a stage that prompts a need for further challenge and change – developing new skills or responsibilities through promotion, or perhaps a need to change direction. Either way, this would require you to disengage (move on from) what you are doing (Box 2.4).

Disengagement

This is Super's final stage of the cycle and it is important to recognise the extent to which careers are built on change. Disengagement is, quite simply, recognition that we leave roles and occupations behind, eventually disengaging from the labour market itself when we cease working.

We hope, of course, that the change we encounter is voluntary, timely and prepared for. However, this is not always the case and the more accustomed we are to reflecting on our strengths, values and interests, articulating our vocational skills and ambitions, and recognising and seizing new opportunities, then the better prepared we are when change happens (Box 2.5).

Possible causes of career change

Estimates vary, but it is widely accepted that careers are more fluid and prone to change than at any time in history. It is likely not only that you will move role many times over the course of your working life but also that you may well change career altogether over the years. Consider just some of the possible causes for career change and how they might influence your journey (Table 2.1).

Box 2.5 Jess

After ten years in occupational therapy, Jess's department is experiencing a major reorganisation. Contracts for service delivery have been tendered and she has the opportunity to either take voluntary redundancy or be redeployed to a new department. Julie is constrained by having family responsibilities, so does not want to move from the area, but is also feeling as if this would be a great opportunity to re-evaluate where her career is.

Exploration for Julie might include:

- Reviewing the last few years: What has she loved about her role? What has frustrated her? If she had the opportunity to change the way she worked, what would change?
- Desktop research to get a sense of what other service providers are established locally.
- Revisit her professional body and consider where there may be opportunities for re-training.
- Arrange some informal meetings with friends and colleagues in other departments (and the new department): What are the opportunities there?
- Review job descriptions (and her Curriculum Vitae [CV] – it needs updating). Thinking about her strengths and interests, are there roles available that really appeal? Are there qualifications or skills that need updating? How can she maximise her chances of a new role?
- Does the offer of voluntary redundancy allow for a more radical change? Would this be a good time to speak to a careers coach to really explore where the next 10 years could lead?

Table 2.1 Causes for career change

Life change	Role change	Market change
• New family • Caring responsibilities • Partner's career change • Injury or ill-health • Changing financial need.	• Promotion or professional development • Departmental or service restructure • Role reorganisation • Specialisation/generalisation, role merging • Personal difficulties in role • Redundancy	• Changes in sector or industry • Technological changes • External competition • Changes to funding streams or contract providers

Throughout your career, awareness of the influences and interests that we have considered in this chapter will help you to make informed decisions. Where change is perhaps unexpected, such an awareness will help you to manage the process with more confidence.

In summary: What do we know? How can this help in considering future chapters?

This chapter was designed to help to frame the idea of developing and managing your career: Career is not something inevitable or accidental, and in order to develop and remain fulfilled in your career you will need to remain aware of the influencing factors that surround you and be prepared to take action to develop new skills and to respond to changing environments.

Super's cycles are just one way of envisioning this process (whilst there are other models that you might find helpful, this example is given to illustrate the process of exploration and planning) and, whilst the external influences of progression, technology and so on are massive, and whilst there will always be influences that cannot be accounted for in your plans, preparedness can help you deal with a lot. Finally, remember that careers can take many forms and shapes!

Potential interview questions in this area
- What motivated you to train in this area?
- Why do you want to work in our organisation?
- What do you know about our organisation?
- What do you think are the key skills required in this role and why are you a good fit?
- What do you expect to be doing in five years' time?
- How will the role contribute to your longer term career goals?
- What are your strengths? What are your weaknesses?

References

Holland JL (1997) Introduction to the theory. In JL Holland, *Making vocational choices: a theory of vocational personalities and work environments*, 3rd edn (pp. 1–15). Odessa, FL: Psychological Assessment Resources.

Hodkinson P (2009) Understanding career decision-making and progression: careership revisited. *Career Research and Development: the NICEC Journal*, **21**:6–7.

Parsons F (1909) *Choosing a Vocation*. Boston, MA: Houghton Mifflin.

Super DE (1953) The dimensions and measurement of vocational maturity. *Teachers College Record*, **57**:151–163.

Super DE (1984) Career and life development. In D. Brown, L. Brooks and Associates (eds), *Career choice and development: Applying contemporary theories to practice* (pp. 192–234). San Francisco, CA: Jossey-Bass.

Super DE (1994) A life-span, life-space perspective on convergence. In ML Savickas and RW Lent (eds), *Convergence in career development theories* (pp. 63–76). Palo Alto, CA: CPP Books.

Super DE, Savickas ML and Super CM (1996) The life-span, life-space approach to careers. In D Brown and L Brooks (eds) *Career choice and development*, 3rd edn). San Francisco, CA: Jossey-Bass.

Yorke M (2004) *Employability in higher education: what it is – what it is not*. Higher Education Academy/ESECT, York, UK.

Chapter 3 **Professionalism**

Rosemarie Mason
School of Health Sciences, University of East Anglia, Norwich, UK

Chapter 1 highlighted the idea that whilst the attainment of competencies is necessary, employability is also reliant on an individual's capacity for self-awareness. The ability to reflect well on one's own values and performance is paramount. Chapter 2 also stressed the importance of understanding one's values and the ways in which they 'fit' with a career path. Chapter 2 and the associated exercises are aimed at helping you to understand who you are. One of the roles you play in life is as a professional person. This chapter will now help to unravel what that means and what the associated responsibilities are. Through having a broader understanding of the concept, you will be better equipped to reflect on your own level of professionalism.

Before we can go on to describe professionalism though, we need to understand what the term 'profession' means.

What is a profession?

Writers have been debating the meaning of the noun 'profession' since the early part of last century. Partly this is because it is a socially constructed concept: that is, it only exists because human beings have created it and talked about it, valued it and used it as a measure to judge people. It is a symbolic thing and an important one but it is constantly evolving and, like the proverbial jellyfish, it is very difficult to pin on a wall. After much academic debate and argument, in 2004 Cruess, Johnston and Cruess

How to Develop Your Healthcare Career: A Guide to Employability and Professional Development, First Edition. Edited by Lisa Taylor.

generated a working definition to assist medical educators in their teaching of professionalism. It is a very good place to start:

> Profession: *An occupation whose core element is work based upon the mastery of a* complex body of knowledge and skills. *It is a* vocation *in which knowledge of some department of* science *or learning or the practice of an* art *founded upon it is used in the* service of others. *Its members are governed by* codes of ethics *and profess a commitment to competence, integrity and morality, altruism, and the promotion of the public good within their domain. These commitments form the basis of a* social contract *between a profession and society, which in return grants the profession a monopoly over the use of its knowledge base, the right to considerable autonomy in practice and the privilege of self-regulation. Professions and their members are* accountable *to those served and to society.*
>
> Cruess, Johnston and Cruess, 2004, p. 75

Let us see if we can tease this out a bit more by looking at individual terms. Firstly, 'social contract'.

What is meant by a 'social contract'

For those professions in the public sector a relationship of mutual dependence has developed between them and the state that employs them. Members of a profession are committed to integrity and are expected to abide by a public service ethic. The state needs professions it can trust to fulfil its social welfare commitments and the professions need the state to allow them an exclusive right to work for it. Professions won this right by persuading the state that competence and trustworthiness could be guaranteed through arduous educational programmes and strong regulatory processes (Wilding, 1982; Freidson, 1994). Under these circumstances the state is prepared to sanction the names of individuals who are certified with the appropriate qualification to appear on an official register: hence, only registered health practitioners can work in the NHS. In return, the state grants the profession a monopoly over the use of its knowledge base, the right to autonomy in practice, the privilege of self-regulation and financial reward (Stevens, 2001; Cruess, Johnston and Cruess, 2004). Under the terms of this contract any deviance from ethical behaviour must be stringently disciplined.

Why is a 'complex body of knowledge and skills' important?

For this we need to look back at history. Skilled expertise and knowledge-based services became significant to society following the Neolithic Revolution (very early history!). When settled agriculture developed and the struggle for survival became more organised, knowledge was unified, which created the opportunity for the cultures of arts and sciences to emerge. Organised religion, philosophy, mathematics, astronomy, medicine and law all began to evolve (Perkin, 1996). The Renaissance (early fifteenth century), the Reformation (early sixteenth century) and the Enlightenment (early seventeenth century) all allowed independent thinkers and innovators to flourish in Europe (Macdonald, 1995; Perkin, 1996). Polyani (1957) called this 'the great transformation'. Knowledge became a source of power, which was then used by occupations to advance their status. For example, in medieval times, law, medicine and the ministry, the classical professions, were under the tutelage of the Church but they were only accessible to a chosen few whose knowledge base was both shrouded in mystery and considered esoteric. Between the eleventh and thirteenth centuries these professions had a closer association with universities (Oxford and Cambridge), where knowledge of Latin distinguished them as 'learned' and still gave them an association with elite society. It was an education based on classical culture rather than practical skill, however (Larson, 1977). Doctors were highly educated and esteemed in society but were very limited in their ability to treat patients effectively (think of purging and leeches). In contrast, people such as tradesmen, scriveners, spectacle makers, apothecaries and barber–surgeons, were associated with and managed by, craft guilds. Their skills were acquired through an apprenticeship with a master (this is where the term 'mastery' comes from). They were very skilled and gradually became respected as society realised the value of their expertise. Thus, Larson (1977) concluded, work could be used to define the place of an individual on a social scale that measured the esteem with which the public held an occupation.

The Industrial Revolution of the eighteenth century onwards introduced enormous changes to the way that people lived. Inventive developments such as piped water, gas and electricity and so on needed to be supplied by people with specific knowledge. A free market had been created and occupations, from engineers to quantity surveyors, proliferated (Perkin, 1996). Freidson (1984) was of the opinion that many people have the ability to learn all of these skills but there is insufficient time in one person's lifetime to undergo the training necessary to learn and sustain competence in every type of skill necessary. Therefore, unless someone lived a very simple life indeed, reliance on the expertise of others had to be established.

This provided the opportunity for groups to improve their status. Larson (1984) outlined the way in which professional leaders realised the importance of knowledge as a form of power and set out to build an ideology of expertise in a defined skill based on the traditional ethic of craftsmanship, emphasising the intrinsic value of work and an ethic of community, emphasising duty. For example, from the sixteenth century, the Royal College of Physicians had monopolised license to practice medicine in London but, elsewhere, medical practitioners from the lower branches, such as apothecaries, were increasingly able to demonstrate that their knowledge of the safe use of drugs was far superior to that of the classically educated doctors. By the eighteenth century, although they had not matched the position of physicians, apothecaries were recognised as genuine medical practitioners and their status had risen. In this way, apothecaries became pharmacists, spectacle makers became optometrists and barbers became surgeons (Larson, 1977). The more closely the knowledge base of emerging professions could be associated with science (emphasising the complex nature of the skill), the better. These developments meant that expertise became a commodity for new professions to use in the employment market (Larson, 1984). For health professions it became necessary to convince the state that they were experts whose competence was superior to others in order to establish a secure footing in NHS employment (Larson, 1984). Although this remains the case today, it is now also recognised that scientific knowledge needs to be applied to unique and complex human problems. There are elements of professional knowledge that cannot be standardised and which must be applied using judgement and artistic interpretation (Schon, 1983): hence, Cruess, Johnston and Cruess' (2004) inclusion of the phrase 'practice of an art' in their definition.

Is vocation still relevant to today's professionals?

The vocational element of being a health professional also has an historical importance. Before the 1930s, virtually all writers on the topic thought that professionalism offered a way of life morally superior to the world of business (Haskell, 1984). It had been assumed that a professional would always act in the best interests of the client, put self-interest aside and provide the highest standard of service (Johnson, 1972). The ideology of specialised knowledge, public service and permanent dedication was considered attractive to people who anchored their identity on such values and, by implication, would be more likely to prove trustworthy in putting the client's interest before their own (Freidson, 1994; Evetts, 2003). It also conveyed the idea that work could have intrinsic value. Finding fulfilment through work is a notion that stems from craftsmanship rather than business ideals. It was in contrast to the norm for the working classes during the industrial revolution, when any work, no matter how unpleasant, was undertaken to avoid starvation, and, therefore, the value was extrinsic (Larson, 1977).

'Vocation' was closely linked with a service ideal, providing it with a religious association. At its most extreme the Florence Nightingale image epitomised the moral pinnacle that must be reached. Traditionally, for example, a nurse:

Must have quelled any desire to enjoy any life which might impinge upon her life as a nurse.

(Alavi and Cattoni, 1995, p. 345).

Today this seems quite extraordinary to ask of anyone.

Subsequently, attention has focused on the idea that, in reality, professionals are just as motivated by self-interest as any other group but the rewards are other forms of 'self-aggrandisement' (status and reputation, for example) rather than financial (Larson, 1977; Haskell, 1984). The image of the selfless professional lingers to a degree (perhaps it is a hope rather than an expectation) but modern reactions to it have been damaged (Freidson, 1994). Governments since the 1980s have questioned the motives behind professional protestations of a service ideal (Foster and Wilding, 2000) whilst Nixon (2003) has reported that since Margaret Thatcher introduced market-driven policies, with a model of private sector managerial professionalism, society has lost sight of the public service ethic.

However, it is also argued that the pursuit of self-interest is not necessarily the antithesis of public interest if it drives the achievement of personal excellence (Haskell, 1984; Evetts, 2003). Since the 1990s there have been calls for a reassessment of the ideals of professionalism to accommodate the changes in the way that professions are organised (Evetts, 2003; Jones and Green, 2006). A study of early-career general practitioners (GPs), for example, revealed that the traditional view of medicine as a vocation, in which a GP would have a therapeutic relationship with a patient from the point of registration until retirement and that they would never be off duty, had been discarded (Jones and Green, 2006). The replacement is a view that medicine is a job with high intrinsic value and that it is important to retain a good work–life balance. Rather than commitment and status in the community, the important moral values now concern the quality of the work undertaken. The implication is that it is more reasonable to expect high-performing excellence from a GP who is able to have a quality home life than from someone who is burnt out from continuous work (Jones and Green, 2006). It is becoming more common for health professionals to expect a right to a private life (Ross *et al.*, 2013). Another study of nursing students also found that the 24 hour per day on-call service had been discarded but there had been benefits in terms of improved person-centred care and more honest communication, so that patients were no longer hidden from the truth about their prognosis, for example (Johnson, Haigh, and Yates-Bolton, 2007). The notions of vocation and altruism are now regarded in a more pragmatic way. Rather than being seen as a detrimental change, the view is that enhanced quality of care is more likely to occur when the expectation of 100% devotion to duty is confined to work hours.

Time for reflection

Where do you stand on your right to a private life? Are there any benefits to your work performance of spending time away from work responsibilities?

Why are codes of ethics so important?

Professional status is a privilege and one that is dependent on the public's belief that professionals are trustworthy (Cruess and Cruess, 1997). Until relatively recently, the expectation of trustworthiness had become so ingrained that both professionals and clients accepted it as the norm (Horobin, 1983). It is fundamental to what individuals are 'professing' to be: people of integrity (Moline, 1986). This claim is usually based on a vow (the Hippocratic Oath, for example) or a code of ethics (Hughes, 1963).

Trust serves two major functions for professions. Firstly, it has long been acknowledged that healthcare professionals have access to privileged information from a vulnerable clientele. Clients will only make disclosures on the understanding that the professional needs to be fully informed in order to resolve the problem and that their confidentiality will be respected. It is right and proper that professionals must be trusted not to abuse such disclosures (Becker, 1977; Hughes, 1981; Moline, 1986). Secondly, the belief that a profession encapsulates a culture that ensures its members will act in the best interests of society is essential as a marketing commodity (Larson, 1977); therefore, trust is necessary to secure a market for employment (Johnson, 1972; Larson, 1977; Wilding, 1982). Trust, embodied within a code of ethics, has become the defining characteristic separating professions from occupations (Moline, 1986; Abbott, 1988; Harrison and Pollitt, 1994).

Time for reflection

How familiar are you with your code of ethics? Could you provide evidence of your trustworthiness?

Greater accountability

It is becoming increasingly important for professionals to be held more accountable. Historically, the relationship between a health professional and client, although patriarchal, has been a fiduciary one. Yet, both the state and public have demonstrated dissatisfaction with professional behaviour lately and there has been a decline in levels of trust (Swick, 2000; Bruhn, 2001; Cruess and Cruess, 2006; Stark et al., 2006; Kell and Owen, 2008). Failure to demonstrate that professions deserve to be trusted has triggered the health reforms of late: Stevens (2001) refers to it as 'antitrust' regulation. Current Government policy in the United Kingdom is aimed at changing the way that health professionals deliver their services. There is now a market basis for health care, which is expected to be delivered with improved, client-focused care. There is an emphasis on more client power and better partnership and dialogue with healthcare providers. *A First Class Service* (Department of Health, 1998) signified for the first time that healthcare professionals must be held accountable for the quality of their care. A strong political interest in ensuring public safety led to new statutory responsibilities for clinical governance supported by structures such as national service frameworks (NSF) and guidelines produced by the National Institute for Health and Care Excellence (NICE). These reforms were only partially successful (Humphrey, 2001). Professional self-regulation, a long-standing reward within the social contract, was considered insufficient to ensure high standards and, therefore, further reforms were needed (Ham, 2004; Klein, 2006).

The Bristol Inquiry (Kennedy, 2001) introduced mechanisms to safeguard the public, such as appraisals to limit the autonomy of practitioners, although the medical profession retained some collegiate self-regulation. The Shipman Inquiry (Smith, 2004) argued that the General Medical Council (GMC) still favoured its members' interests over those of the public. The Government therefore proposed changes to the regulatory framework for healthcare professions (Department of Health, 2006), including a radical transformation of the GMC's remit, removing its judicial role, control of medical education and undermining self-regulation (Klein, 2006). Alongside this were proposals for the revalidation of nurses and health professionals, encompassing fitness to practice and continuing professional development (CPD). In 2007, the Government published a White Paper entitled *Trust, Assurance and Safety* (Department of Health, 2007). This proposed changes to the regulatory framework for health professionals in the United Kingdom, highlighting the importance of trust within the relationship between professionals, their clientele and the Government. More recent legislation, including *High Quality Care for All* (Department of Health, 2008), the *Health and Social Care Act* (Department of Health, 2012), and The *NHS Constitution* (Department of Health, 2013), all emphasise increased accountability for the quality of service, more effective performance management and greater acknowledgement of the primacy of the client. This redefinition of the role of clients, as consumers, and healthcare workers, as providers of health care, is significant. The intent is to bring equity into the relationship between the two, in contrast to traditional professional practice where the authoritative professional expert has primacy.

Professions are held to account for their actions through their regulatory bodies: in the case of allied health professions, the Health and Care Professions Council (HCPC). The HCPC's responsibility includes publication of best practice guidelines, approval of qualifying courses, registration and monitoring of qualified professionals, and disciplinary processes for the 16 professions they regulate (HCPC, 2012). Every two years registrants are required to sign a declaration of their continued fitness to practice and a percentage of them are audited more closely. The Nursing and Midwifery

Council has agreed a model for launching a revalidation process by December 2015. This will require nurses and midwives to revalidate every three years; to meet a required number of hours of practice and learning activity based on a revised code of professional conduct, to undertake reflection and to obtain confirmation of their continuing fitness to practise from someone well placed to comment (Nursing and Midwifery Council, 2013).

Despite the number of regulatory processes there has been an inescapable change in the public perception of healthcare professions' capacity to deliver their contractual obligations. Any regulatory framework takes into account the idea that confidence in the trustworthiness of healthcare workers must be justified. Trust is now becoming something that is legislatively imposed rather than being inherent within the culture of the profession itself. Healthcare may be market driven but this does not inevitably lead to the exclusion of trustworthiness: some trades people have been very successful in earning respect from their clientele. Bruhn (2001) suggests that health professionals should anticipate and adapt to the way in which health care now operates and aim to re-establish trust as a professional characteristic. Of course, placing trust in another person requires a degree of dependence on the service provider, which may not sit well with the notion of greater client power. However, there is evidence to suggest that traditional ethical values associated with professional practice are still held in high regard by clients (Cruess, Johnston and Cruess, 2004), suggesting there is room for mediation.

A research report published by the Health and Care Professions Council (HCPC, 2015) argues that regulation at a microlevel has disadvantages in that behaviours are enforced rather than being something that people naturally want to do because it is part of who they are. For too long there has been a focus entirely on measurable competency when appraising the work of health and social care practitioners. The call is for a renewed emphasis on professionalism as a value-based (ethical) concept and we need to develop in ourselves, things that cannot be measured quantitatively (compassion/empathy etc.).

So far we have tried to explain why a definition of a profession is important. You may have noticed that a lot of it is concerned with the way professions are organised and how people act within them. In the next section we will explain the link between being a professional and an individual's sense of self (having a professional identity).

Why is professional identity important?

It has been noted that the domain of social identity has been subjected to a wealth of theorisation but the work of sociologist Erving Goffman (1922–1982) continues to have currency for research about professional identity (Atkinson and Housley, 2003). Goffman built on the work of philosopher and sociologist, George Mead to explore the social organisation of professional identity. He was particularly interested in the relationship between the psychological preoccupation with self and the ways through which identity is formed by social processes and accomplished through interactions with others (Atkinson and Housley, 2003). Goffman's concept of identity is multilayered and concerns what the individual says, thinks, imagines and what the person 'is' (Atkinson and Housley, 2003). He argued that professional status involves more than achieving a prestigious place in society. It also concerns a public presentation of oneself as being close to commonly respected societal values and, therefore, allows individuals to adopt a highly regarded sense of self (Goffman, 1969). Certainly this fits in with the early sociologists' view of the professions' close approximation to high moral values.

Goffman established the idea that professional identity can be generated through rituals that occur within interactions (Atkinson and Housley, 2003). When clients expect professionals to be imbued with trust and that expectation is fulfilled, then the idea that trust is an important professional characteristic is perpetuated (Hughes, 1981). The ritualistic offering and receiving of trusting actions highlights the ethicality of the professional person. Thus, the manifestation of a trusting relationship is one of the ways through which individuals can 'perform' their professionalism and, therefore, confirm their identity. Bruhn (2001) noted that the opportunity to be 'good' by doing good is what motivates people to become health profession-als and permits a positive answer to the question, 'Can I be proud of who I appear to be?' Being a professional is closely bounded with who a person 'is'. As Moline (1986) reported, if a plumber loses his or her job it might be annoying but if the same thing happened to a doctor it would be catastrophic, because the foundation for that individual's self-belief has been removed.

It is therefore important for health and social care practitioners to become confident in their sense of self as a professional person and to have the necessary resilience to remain committed to ethical ideals whatever the cir-cumstances. Where an individual's professional identity stems from common values, this also means that members of the same group share work practices, procedures, the ways in which they perceive the knowledge base and solu-tions to problems as well as views on interactions with clients (Evetts, 2003). In this way, each individual is responsible for contributing to the way in which the whole profession is perceived.

Time for reflection
Think about that phrase: 'Can I be proud of who I appear to be?' How would you answer this question? What values does your profession uphold and do you share them? How do your clientele know that you have these values?

Let us now turn our attention to professionalism. To start: What is the difference between 'profession' and 'professionalism'? The suffix 'ism' is used to convert the noun (profession) into an active noun. So, in 'doing' professionalism you are 'being' a profession.

Professionalism concerns knowledge and skills (competence) and also values, beliefs and attitudes, which drive behaviours (conduct). As we have seen, some of these characteristics are inherent in individuals who choose professional careers. The next section explains how these are further developed in education.

Learning professionalism

Many authors have identified the importance of the educational curriculum in developing professionalism in doctors (Shapiro, Rucker and Robitshek, 2006; O'Sullivan and Toohey, 2008; van Mook *et al.*, 2009a; Passi *et al.*, 2010) and to some extent amongst allied health professionals (Kasar and Muscari, 2000; Lindquist *et al.*, 2006). Medical schools have previously focused their assessment strategies on knowledge and skills acquisition (Stark *et al.*, 2006). In the United Kingdom, the General Medical Council now recommends that attitudinal learning objectives should be given equal importance in the curriculum to knowledge and skills objectives (GMC, 2009). For example, outcome 3 of the 'Outcomes and standards for undergraduate medical education' (page 25) concerns the doctor as a professional. Graduates must behave according to ethical principles, including being polite, considerate, trustworthy and honest. They must respect all patients and colleagues and recognize the rights and the equal value of all people (GMC, 2009).

Traditionally, it had been assumed that health students would absorb the elements of professionalism through socialisation. This remains important but it is now recognised that the concept must also be explicitly taught (Cruess and Cruess, 2006) and assessed (van Mook *et al.*, 2009b, 2009c). Studies within the medical profession suggest that learning about professionalism should take into account cognitive (factual) knowledge of the topic. Students must be informed about theoretical underpinnings and understand what professionalism is. They can then learn the behavioural components, which might include performance and skills acquisition (Hodges *et al.*, 2011). In addition, specific character traits, attitudes and values need to be fostered (van Mook *et al.*, 2009b; Wearn *et al.*, 2010). Learning and assessment, therefore, require a combination of approaches that address each of these components. Chapters 1 and 2 have shown that employers are not just looking for skilled competence but also the values, beliefs and attitudes that harmonise with those of their organisation.

Cruess and Cruess (2006) have argued that situated learning theory is the most appropriate way to develop professionalism in students. Briefly, this theory has a fundamental tenet that learning should be embedded in authentic activities. It is important to provide students with a definition of professionalism and then give opportunities for long-term experience and reflection on performance in different contexts and situations, particularly in practice, and to offer constructive feedback (van Mook *et al.*, 2009b; Goldie, 2013). Through these means, knowledge can be transformed from the theoretical to the useable and useful (Cruess and Cruess, 2006). Principal among the factors to consider when using situated learning theory is a stipulation that the educational institution must agree on both the definition and description of professionalism and that these must be consistently portrayed throughout the educational process. The definition provided by Cruess, Johnston and Cruess (2004) at the opening of this chapter is a good one. We will now consider a description of professionalism.

For the benefit of the medical profession, three organisations – the European Federation of Internal Medicine, the American College of Physicians and American Society of Internal Medicine and the American Board of Internal Medicine – developed a 'Charter on Medical Professionalism'. This charter was written in response to a perceived need to make explicit the ideals to which doctors throughout the world are committed (Charter on Medical Professionalism, 2002). This was a global exercise that seems to have reached an agreement on the responsibilities required of physicians. Notwithstanding that there is some continuing debate about describing professionalism (van Mook *et al.*, 2009c), the School of Health Sciences (HSC) at the University of East Anglia (UEA) used this work to inform the development of its own 'Professionalism Charter', the details of which have been published elsewhere (Mason *et al.*, 2012a, 2012b). The UEA has described professionalism as a collection of nineteen values, attitudes skills and aspects of knowledge (collectively termed 'responsibilities') organised within five concepts (Table 3.1). The Professionalism Charter is used as a framework to inform all teaching and assessment of professionalism for a range of health and social care students.

Students are expected to accumulate evidence of their growth in respect to each of the responsibilities within their continuing professional development portfolio. They have regular voluntary meetings with a personal advisor and one obligatory meeting at the end of each academic year. The purpose of this meeting is to review the student's progress related to the responsibilities within the charter. The style of the meeting is one of mentorship in which personal advisors are expected to guide the student through their personal journey towards professionalism. Evaluations to date have shown that the Professionalism Charter is an effective mechanism through which to guide

Table 3.1 The University of East Anglia Professionalism Charter. Adapted from UEA 2012

Professionalism concept	Associated responsibilities
Moral and ethical values	Honesty and integrity
	Empathy and compassion
	Altruism and respect for others
	Trustworthiness and dependability
Commitment to improve	Supervision
	Reflective practice
	Self-awareness
Managing self and others	Organisation
	Effective verbal communication
	Effective written communication
Clinical competence	Initiative
	Clinical reasoning
	Competence
	Judgement
Personal accountability	Responsibility
	Cooperation
	Confidentiality
	Professional presentation
	Maintain appropriate
	relationships with service users

professional growth (Mason *et al.*, 2014). It is our belief that although the specific skills required for clinical competence will be different for each profession, the concepts of moral and ethical values, commitment to improve, managing self and others and personal accountability are common to any health professional.

A word about social media

In theory, the tenets of professionalism that we have talked about should apply in all circumstances, regardless of the context or situation, and that includes the use of social media. There is no difference between real life and online professional identity (Kaczmarczyk, 2013). The use of social media is a fixed part of everyday life and if used responsibly has the potential for good in health care (Reed *et al.*, 2013). However, a number of studies have shown that health professionals do not always realise how easy it is for them to compromise professionalism when using networking sites such as Facebook. This is likely to become more of a concern as the liberal sharing of digital information develops further (Kaczmarczyk, 2013). Professional organisations publish guidelines on the use of social media but these are often lengthy and difficult to locate and not necessarily written by people who are most familiar with the technology (Osman, Wardle and Caesar, 2012). One of the more accessible links to guidance from the General Medical Council is: http://www.gmc-uk.org/guidance/ethical_guidance/21186.asp

Many health professionals have dissonant views about what is appropriate online and in real life (Osman, Wardle and Caesar, 2012; Ross, 2013; Kaczmarczyk, 2013). Their online identity is seen as different to their professional identity. Osman, Wardle and Caesar's (2012) study found that 67% of registrars and doctors believe that there are photographs of themselves on Facebook that could compromise their own professionalism and 88% of medical students in their sample had seen colleagues behaving unprofessionally on Facebook. Whilst younger people (students) were most likely to activate privacy settings, more senior doctors were not careful in restricting access to their posted information (Osman, Wardle and Caesar, 2012). The types of unprofessional conduct that have been noted on social media sites include (Reed *et al.*, 2013; Kaczmarczyk, 2013; Cunningham, 2014; Kleebauer, 2014):

- Failure to activate privacy settings.
- Inappropriate communication (including 'friending') with patients or between educators and students.
- Misrepresentation of credentials.
- Breaches of confidentiality.
- Compromising photographs (involving excessive drinking or overt sexual behaviour).
- Use of discriminatory or foul language.
- Disparaging remarks about an organisation, patients or colleagues.

There have been calls for 'e-professionalism' rules to be established (Cain and Romanelli, 2009) but, in truth, they would be no different to the rules that already exist. It is wise for us all to remember that a professional lapse occurring in the workplace would be an uncomfortable experience; imagine the magnitude of the same error if it was played out to a global audience.

Summary

This chapter has provided a sociological explanation of the concepts of 'profession' and 'professionalism'. It is a topic that is continually evolving in response to political, organisational and individual events. It is closely linked to an individual's sense of self. That being the case, it is important to be aware of one's own position and those of the external agencies influencing the concept to ensure harmony between your own values, attitudes and behaviours and those embedded in the career of your choice. The next chapter will enhance your understanding of how this kind of knowledge may be documented within a framework of continuing professional development.

Potential interview questions in this area

• How might you respond to a member of staff who tells you that it is acceptable to take case notes home to write them up?
• How might you show compassion in your work?
• How important is it to continue to improve your practice?
• How can you demonstrate responsibility in the workplace?
• Why is trustworthiness important in the workplace?
• What would be your response if you spotted unprofessional behaviour by a colleague on Facebook?

References

Abbott A (1988) *The system of professions: an essay on the division of expert labour.* Chicago, IL: The University of Chicago Press.

Alavi C and Cattoni J (1995) Good nurse, bad nurse… *Journal of Advanced Nursing,* **21**:344–349.

Atkinson P and Housley W (2003) *Interactionism.* London: Sage.

Becker HS (1977) *Sociological work. Method and substance.* New Brunswick, NJ: Transaction Books.

Bruhn JG (2001) Being good and doing good: The culture of professionalism in the health professions. *Health Care Manager,* **19**(4):47–58.

Cain J and Romanelli F (2009) A new paradigm for a digital age. *Currents in Pharmacy Teaching and Learning,* **1**:66–70.

Charter on Medical Professionalism (2002) Medical professionalism in the new millennium: a physicians' charter. *The Lancet,* **359**:520–522.

Cruess SR and Cruess RL. (1997) Professionalism must be taught. *British Medical Journal,* **315**:1674–1677.

Cruess RL and Cruess SR (2006) Teaching professionalism: General principles. *Medical Teacher,* **28**(3):205–208.

Cruess RC, Johnston S and Cruess RL (2004) "Profession": A working definition for medical educators. *Teaching and Learning in Medicine,* **16**(1):74–76.

Cunningham A (2014) Social media and medical professionalism. *Medical Education,* **48**:110–112.

Department of Health (1998) *A first class service: Quality in the new NHS.* London: HMSO.

Department of Health (2006) *The regulation of the non-medical healthcare professions: a review by the Department of Health.* Gateway reference: 6856. London: HMSO.

Department of Health (2007) *Trust, assurance and safety – The regulation of health professionals in the 21st Century.* Cm 7013. London: HMSO.

Department of Health (2008) *High quality care for all*. Gateway reference: 10106. London: HMSO.

Department of Health (2012) *Health and Social Care Act*. Retrieved from https://www.gov.uk/government/publications/health-and-social-care-act-2012-fact-sheets (last accessed 5 August 2015).

Department of Health (2013) *The NHS Constitution for England*. Retrieved from https://www.gov.uk/government/publications/the-nhs-constitution-for-england (last accessed 5 August 2015).

Evetts. J (2003) The sociological analysis of professionalism: Occupational change in the modern world. *International Sociology*, **18**(2):395–414.

Foster P and Wilding P (2000) Whither welfare professionalism? *Social Policy and Administration*, **34**(2):143–159.

Freidson E (1984) Are professions necessary? In TL Haskell (ed.) *The authority of experts* (pp. 3–27). Bloomington, IN: Indiana University Press.

Freidson E (1994) *Professionalism re-born. Theory, prophecy and policy*. Cambridge: Polity Press.

(GMC) General Medical Council (2009) *Tomorrow's doctors: Recommendations on undergraduate medical education*. http://www.gmc-uk.org/Tomorrow_s_Doctors_1214.pdf_48905759.pdf (last accessed 3 September 2015).

Goffman E (1969, reprinted 1990) *The presentation of self in everyday life*. Middlesex, UK: Penguin Books.

Goldie J (2013) Assessment of professionalism: A consolidation of current thinking. *Medical Teacher*, **35**:e952–e956.

Ham C (2004) *Health Policy in Britain*, 5th edn (revised and updated). New York: Palgrave Macmillan.

Harrison S and Pollitt C (1994) *Controlling health professionals: the future of work and organization in the National Health Service*. Buckingham, UK: Open University Press.

Haskell TL (1984) *Professionalism versus capitalism. The authority of experts*. Bloomington, IN: Indiana University Press.

Health and Care Professions Council (2012) *Why your HCPC registration matters*. Retrieved from http://www.hcpc-uk.org/publications/ (last accessed 5 August 2015).

HCPC (2015) *Preventing small problems from becoming big problems in health and care*. Retrieved from http://www.hcpc-uk.org/publications/ (last accessed 5 August 2015).

Hodges BD, Ginsburgh S, Cruess R, *et al*. (2011) Assessment of professionalism: Recommendations from the Ottawa 2010 Conference. *Medical Teacher*, **33**:354–363.

Horobin G (1983) Professional mystery: The maintenance of charisma in general medical practice. In R Dingwall and P Lewis (eds) *The Sociology of the professions, lawyers, doctors and others*. London: Macmillan Press.

Hughes EC (1963) *The Professions*. Daedalus, **92**(4):655–668.

Hughes EC (1981) *Men and their work*. Westport, CT: Greenwood Press.

Humphrey C (2001) Six policy briefing papers prepared for the Bristol Royal Infirmary Public Inquiry. In *Annex B of the Inquiry Report Learning from Bristol: the report of the public inquiry into children's heart surgery at the Bristol Royal Infirmary 1984–1995*. Command Paper: CM52 07. London: The Stationery Office Limited.

Johnson TJ (1972) *Professions and power.* London: Macmillan Press.

Johnson M, Haigh C and Yates-Bolton N (2007) Valuing altruism and honesty in nursing students: A two-decade replication study. *Journal of Advanced Nursing,* **57**(4):366–374.

Jones L and Green J (2006) Shifting discourses of professionalism: A case study of general practitioners in the United Kingdom. *Sociology of Health and Illness,* **28**(7):927–950.

Kaczmarczyk JM, Chuang A, Dugoff L *et al.* (2013) e-Professionalism: A New Frontier in Medical Education. *Teaching and Learning in Medicine,* **25**(2):165–170.

Kasar J and Muscari ME (2000) A conceptual model for the development of professional behaviours in occupational therapists. *Canadian Journal of Occupational Therapy,* **67**(1):43–50.

Kell C and Owen G (2008) Physiotherapy as a profession: Where are we now? *International Journal of Therapy and Rehabilitation,* **15**(4):158–164.

Kennedy (2001) *Bristol Royal Infirmary Public Inquiry: Report Learning from Bristol: the report of the public inquiry into children's heart surgery at the Bristol Royal Infirmary 1984–1995.* Command Paper: CM5207. London: HMSO.

Kleebauer A (2014) When trouble can be just a click away. *Nursing Standard,* **28**(49):20–21.

Klein P (2006) *The new politics of the NHS.* Abingdon, UK: Radcliffe Publishing Ltd.

Larson MS (1977) *The rise of professionalism: A sociological analysis.* London: University of California Press.

Larson MS (1984) The production of expertise and the constitution of expert power. In TL Haskell (ed.) *The authority of experts* (pp. 28–80). Bloomington, IN: Indiana University Press.

Lindquist I, Engardt M, Garnham L *et al.* (2006) Physiotherapy students' professional identity on the edge of working life. *Medical Teacher,* **28**(3):270–276.

Macdonald KM (1995) *The sociology of the professions.* London:Sage Publications.

Mason R, Vitkovitch J, Jepson J and Lambert R (2012) Having the Conversation. *RCSLT Bulletin,* September 18–19.

Mason R, Jepson J, Vitkovitch J and Lambert R (2012) Instilling professionalism in education. *OTnews,* October 30–31.

Mason R, Vitkovitch J, Lambert R and Jepson J (2014) Knowing about and performing professionalism: Developing professionalism in interprofessional healthcare education. *International Journal of Practice-Based Learning in Health and Social Care,* **2**(1):96–107.

Moline JN (1986) Professionals and professions: A philosophical examination of an ideal. *Social Science Medicine,* **22**(5):501–508.

Nixon J (2003) *What is Theory?* Keynote address delivered at the 'Putting theory into practice: occupational therapy as a complex intervention' conference. College of Occupational Therapists, 17 September 2003, London.

Nursing and Midwifery Council (2013) *Revalidation strategy and model for consultation agreed by Council.* http://www.nmc-uk.org/Nurses-and-midwives/Revalidation/Key-revalidation-dates/ (last accessed 5 August 2015).

Osman A, Wardle A and Caesar R (2012) Online professionalism and Facebook – Falling through the generation gap. *Medical Teacher,* **34**:e549–e556.

O'Sullivan AJ and Toohey SM (2008) Assessment of professionalism in undergraduate medical students. *Medical Teacher*, **30**(3):280–286.

Passi, V. Doug M, Peile E *et al.* (2010) Developing medical professionalism in future doctors: a systematic review. *International Journal of Medical Education*, **1**:19–29.

Perkin H (1996) *The third revolution. Professional elites in the modern world.* London: Routledge.

Polyani K (1957) *The great transformation.* Boston, MA: Beacon Press.

Reed D, Mueller PS, Hafferty FW and Brennan MD (2013) Contemporary issues in medical professionalism. Challenges and opportunities. *Minnesota Medicine*, **96**(11):44–47.

Ross S (2013) 'I have the right to a private life': Medical students'views about professionalism in a digital world. *Medical Teacher*, **35**(10):826–831.

Schon DA (1983) *The reflective practitioner: How professionals think in action.* Aldershot, UK: Ashgate Arena.

Shapiro J, Rucker L and Robitshek D (2006) Teaching the art of doctoring: an innovative medical student elective. *Medical Teacher*, **28**(1):30–35.

Smith J (2004) *Fifth Report – Safeguarding Patients: Lessons from the Past – Proposals for the Future:* Norwich, UK: HMSO.

Stark P, Roberts C, Newble D and Bax N (2006) Discovering professionalism through guided reflection. *Medical Teacher*, **28**(1):e25–e31

Stevens RA (2001) Public roles for the medical profession in the United States: Beyond theories of decline and fall. *The Milbank Quarterly*, **79**(3):327–353.

Swick HM (2000) Toward a normative definition of medical professionalism. *Academic Medicine*, **75**(6):612–616.

van Mook WNKA, de Grave WS, van Luijk SJ *et al.* (2009a) Training and learning professionalism in the medical school curriculum: Current considerations. *European Journal of Internal Medicine*, **20**:e96–e100 (www.elsevier.com/locate/ejim; last accessed 5 August 2015).

van Mook WNKA, van Luijk SJ, O'Sullivan H *et al.* (2009b) General considerations regarding assessment of professional behavior. *European Journal of Internal Medicine*, **20**:e90–e95 (www.elsevier.com/locate/ejim; last accessed 5 August 2015).

van Mook WNKA, Scheltus J, O'Sullivan H *et al.* (2009c) The concepts of professionalism and professional behaviour: Conflicts in both definition and learning outcomes. *European Journal of Internal Medicine*, **20**:e85–e89 (www.elsevier.com/locate/ejim; last accessed 5 August 2015).

Wearn A, Wilson H, Hawken SJ *et al.* (2010) In search of professionalism: implications for medical education. *Journal of the New Zealand Medical Association*, **123**(1314) [online].

Wilding P (1982) *Professional power and social welfare.* London: Routledge.

Chapter 4 Continuing professional development (CPD)

James Gazzard
School of Health Sciences, University of East Anglia, Norwich, UK

Introduction

Global health and social care economies are affected more than ever by rapid – and frequently unpredictable – political, economic, sociological, technological, environmental and legal change. No single registered health professional can confidently forecast the future, other than to say that it will be subject to profound upheaval.

The commitment to remain open minded, continually learn and apply that learning – across a career that for many professionals now entering the workforce may last for around half a century – for the benefit of service users will be one of the key difference between individuals and organisations that succeed and those that do not. The stakes around continuing professional development (CPD) are high, therefore, for patients, the careers of professionals that care for them, and the employers of these health and care professionals. An effective approach to CPD is one of a set of critical success factors that must be addressed by health and care professionals who are intent on driving significant, valuable and potentially radical changes, to ensure that the health and well-being of the communities they serve are improved.

It is vital that all health and care professionals have far more than a cursory understanding of CPD, an understanding, in fact, that extends well beyond the basics. For example, an understanding of the 'amount' of CPD required over a certain time period to maintain their registration if they are to maximise their job satisfaction, respond to the needs of employers, deliver exceptional patient care – and ultimately optimise their career-long employability.

How to Develop Your Healthcare Career: A Guide to Employability and Professional Development, First Edition. Edited by Lisa Taylor.
© 2016 John Wiley & Sons, Ltd. Published 2016 by John Wiley & Sons, Ltd.

Objectives

This chapter seeks to demystify CPD for those who are current pre-registration health and care students or who are registered practitioners in the early part of their career.

Outline guidance on how to plan and enact a meaningful CPD portfolio that results in the transfer of learning into practice is provided later on in this chapter and is deliberately not a 'painting by numbers' guide to CPD. Sadly, CPD is conceived of by some professionals and their employers as a chore to be completed, or a 'tick box' exercise, where the minimum to achieve continued registration or revalidation is considered satisfactory. Those professionals with an understanding of how to think about, plan and execute an approach to CPD that underpins their growth as a provider of exceptional care will be far better placed to take ownership of their career trajectory, and by association enjoy a more fulfilled career. Consequently, the chapter will help the reader to understand:

- What CPD is, and its link to employability.
- The types of learning that underpins the most effective types of CPD.
- The variety of forms CPD takes, particularly the importance of a CPD mix that maximises the use of informal (work-based learning) and formal educational programmes.
- Levels of CPD, specifically credit-bearing and non-credit-bearing CPD.
- An approach to judging the impact of CPD, specifically whether learning has been transferred to practice.
- How to overcome the barriers to accessing CPD, particularly limited time and funding.
- A practical outline guide to planning and undertaking effective CPD.

It should be noted that whilst the chapter is relevant to all health and care disciplines, it does not exhaustively list the procedures required by healthcare professional regulatory bodies to complete their individual CPD requirements. This is because these requirements vary over time and are subject to change (e.g. forthcoming revalidation requirements). Up-to-date details of the amount (if specified, in hours or perhaps as CPD points) of CPD required over a certain period, the types of CPD permitted in a portfolio and the forms of evidence required to document their completion can be found on the web site of the relevant regulatory body. It is advisable to check the CPD pages of your regulatory body at least a couple of times each year to ensure you are aware of any proposed changes (remembering that if you work internationally the requirements will vary quite considerably from what you may have previously experienced). Usually, CPD requirements will be clearly specified; if not, a call or e-mail to their helpdesk will normally result in a quick answer to specific queries.

Throughout this chapter we will consider CPD as a vital pillar of your career development and employability, alongside regularly practicing as a clinician and the mandatory training that your employer will require you to complete.

The terminology of CPD

The continuing professional development field is awash with terminology, an alphabet soup of abbreviations. Throughout this chapter the term continuing professional development (CPD) will be used. However, there are a plethora of variants, including continuing education (CE), continuing professional education (CPE), continuing professional and personal development (CPPD), post-registration education, learning beyond registration, professional education, lifelong learning – and others are emerging all of time.

It is interesting and important to note that the word '*training*' is absent from most of the current nomenclature pertaining to professional development. This may be because training has historically implied the acquisition of a rather rigid and contained set of skills to perform a specific set of tasks, without necessarily understanding the underpinning theory. In a rapidly changing world there is a perceived danger that trained skills may well become outmoded and the trained individual unable to adapt to their new circumstances.

However, some graduate employers now claim that university students are '*overeducated*' in the underlying theory but '*under trained*' in the workplace application of their knowledge (Archer and Davison, 2008). This highlights the need for balance between knowledge acquisition and the capacity, and necessary opportunities, to apply that learning. Any approach to CPD that is unbalanced – with a continued overemphasis on either pure education or narrow task-focused training – is unlikely be successful in the medium-to-long term.

A definition of CPD

The Health and Care Professions Council in the United Kingdom (HCPC) defines CPD as:

> '*a range of learning activities through which health care professionals maintain and develop throughout their career to ensure that they retain their capacity to practice safely, effectively and legally within their evolving scope of practice*'

The care sector organisation Skills for Care defines CPD as:

'planned learning and development activity that develops, maintains or extends knowledge, skills, understanding or performance'

The American Nurses Association (ANA) defines CPD as:

'a lifelong process of active participation by nurses in learning activities that assist in developing the maintaining their continuing competence, enhance their professional practice, and support achievement of their career goals'

These definitions share some similarities. All consider CPD to be a *process*. In this chapter we will explore this process, so that early-career professionals can optimise their approach to CPD.

Each of the three illustrative definitions places the *responsibility* for undertaking CPD directly on to the healthcare professional; ultimately, this is unarguable, one essential requirement of professionalism is to demonstrate a personal commitment to learn and appropriately apply that learning to practice. However, it is important that this should not be confused with CPD being an individual and isolated process. For example, learning in groups or teams (e.g. a group of colleagues who work together) is often an effective way of engaging with CPD. Furthermore, employers should ensure that the CPD of their employees joins up to address important strategic targets.

Significantly, each of the definitions makes reference, explicit or implied, to the link between CPD and *patient safety*. They each suggest that CPD is a critical part of ensuring that health and social care professionals are safe to practice. CPD is an important part of ensuring that avoidable errors and adverse events are avoided and that, more broadly, CPD plays a vital role in ensuring service users are provided with the best available and most contemporary treatments, care and advice.

Likewise, as you would expect, they each stress the notions of career-long 'continuing' learning, tacitly implying the need for *regular engagement* with CPD. The centrality of maintaining previously acquired competencies and professional development, growth and improvement are also common elements to the definitions.

The HCPC definition, as might be anticipated from a regulatory body, mentions the requirement to work within the *law*. A vital consideration particularly, for example, as the role boundaries of health professionals continue to grow and increase in complexity.

All of these components of the definitions are important to informing our understanding of what CPD should be about as early career practitioners. However, it could be argued that some important elements are missing or are underemphasised, particularly for early-career practitioners seeking to maximise their employability.

Whilst the Skills for Care definition highlights the need for *planning* of the CPD agenda, perhaps insufficient emphasis is placed by the definitions on the need for professionals to take stock – by regularly looking forwards and backwards – at their CPD mix. Clearly, practitioners must be prepared for their day-to-day job role in the short term. However, they must also consider the knowledge, skills and attributes they are likely to require in future roles – linking their CPD agenda to the career trajectory to which they aspire. These varied requirements suggest that any meaningful CPD mix is likely to contain an assortment of different types of learning opportunities.

None of the definitions describes what types of CPD should be undertaken. We shall explore this in more detail later in the chapter.

In addition to personal responsibility, however, CPD should be considered as a partnership of learning between the healthcare professional and their line manager, which, in turn, is aligned to the priorities of the employing organisation. The line manager's and the employer's roles are essential in the sense that they must support the professional to deploy and develop their learning in the workplace to ensure that patients benefit optimally from the investment in CPD.

Surprisingly, given the requirement by most regulatory bodies to keep appropriate records of CPD undertaken, it is interesting that none of the definitions specifically set out this requirement. It is essential that all students and graduates familiarise themselves with the CPD record keeping required by their regulatory body, and put in place an approach to respond to this need.

The ANA definition also extends to link CPD to the achievement of career goals. This may encompass goals such as achieving specialist qualifications, or perhaps hoped for promotions to increased levels of responsibility and seniority. However, it is possible to extend this further to consider the role CPD can play in job role and career satisfaction. The personal and professional fulfilment that can be obtained through making the transition from novice to expert in a field of interest, or sustainably improving the performance of a clinical area can, in part, be unlocked by well-designed and well-timed CPD programmes. The virtuous circle of job satisfaction leading to higher workplace performance and, hence, greater employability is clear.

Motivations to engage with CPD

It is important to consider your own motivations for engaging with CPD. The vast majority of health and care professionals are positively motivated by maintaining a high standard of professional competence. Also, there is a positive peer pressure amongst professionals that drives them to want to present a professional image, and enhance their professional status in the field.

Other drivers to engage with CPD are economic. At one level, registered professionals must be able to evidence their CPD activities to maintain their registered status. Beyond that CPD is an important platform on which to achieve promotion and higher levels of financial reward.

Time for reflection

Take the time to talk with colleagues or peers to discuss your motivations for engaging with CPD

The precursors of effective CPD

A considerable amount of research has been undertaken in a range of disciplines to determine the range of factors that determine whether the learner is able to transfer their learning from CPD into practice (Blume *et al.*, 2010). An awareness of these precursors can help to learners to understand how the process of CPD can be optimised. The factors can be divided into three groups

1. *Characteristics of the learner*
   A range of studies suggest that the learner's cognitive ability (e.g. the learner's ability to understand complex ideas, adapt to new environments and learn from experience), their level of self-efficacy (the learner's perceived judgment of their ability to perform a given task), personal motivation (e.g. their intensity, direction and determination of effort to learn) and their sense of whether the CPD has a high utility (i.e. the CPD is relevant in terms of its content and its link to their job role) influence learning.

2. *Design of the CPD*
   In order to encourage learning transfer into practice it is suggested that CPD should display the characteristics of behavioural modelling. Behavioural modelling is a set of learning principles that includes clearly defined explanations of the behaviours to be learned, opportunities for learners to practice new skills and clear feedback on their learning. It is also suggested that CPD that contains 'error management' is effective in encouraging transfer of learning to practice; error management allows learners to understand, as part of their learning, what can go wrong and how to correct the problem (e.g. using simulation as part of the learning). Additionally, it is proposed that the learning environment should be realistic; either on-the-job learning, or in environments that simulate realistic aspects of the work environment.

3. *Workplace environment*

The work environment in which the learner attempts to apply their newly learnt knowledge, skills and attitudes is a critical factor. The 'transfer climate' depends on whether, for example, learners are encouraged to use their learning at work, peers and managers provide positive feedback for the application of the learning and learners may be rewarded in various ways (e.g. praise, more responsibility, financially) for the use of their learning as part of their job role. Supervisor and peer support to deploy the learning is vital; for example, before the CPD event supervisors should set achievable goals for how the learning will be used at work, and after training supervisors should set short-term and long-term goals for applying the new competencies in the workplace. A lack of management support is cited in many studies as a frequent barrier to the transfer of learning to work. As a related observation, learners need to be provided with time and frequent opportunities to use the learning at work, preferably very shortly after the CPD event. Supervisors should also make time to engage the learners in feedback sessions to debrief them on their application of the learning.

Given that research informs us of the critical ingredients of the recipe for successful CPD, we can use this to our advantage. For example, you should consider whether a CPD course is really relevant to your learning needs (i.e. does it have a high utility?), or if a CPD course contains opportunities to practise new skills or whether it is purely didactic, such as 'chalk and talk' lectures (e.g. there is evidence purely instructional CPD does not lead to transfer of learning to practice), and whether you are able to involve your line manager in the planning of your CPD agenda to ensure you will be supported to have repeated opportunities to refine your learning in the workplace shortly after the CPD programme.

Time for reflection

Consider a recent CPD learning activity you have undertaken. Based on the identified precursors for successful CPD consider the ways in which the learning could have been more effectively designed and transferred to practice.

Types of CPD: What counts as CPD?

It is not an overstatement to say that CPD opportunities are everywhere. It would certainly be a mistake to think that CPD can only occur in a formal learning setting, such as a classroom at a university. Formal learning such as a Masters degree can be a very important aspect of career-wide learning but the informal learning that takes place every day at work, for example from observing senior colleagues or receiving feedback from your line manager, can be core components of learning to be a highly effective practitioner.

As many health and care professions have moved towards becoming graduate-only, an emphasis and value has been placed on formal learning, such as accredited university programmes. These accredited programmes generally incorporate a formal assessment, such as a written exam or objective structured clinical examination (OSCE). Accordingly, each learner can be shown to have reached the required standard and certification will be provided to reassure current or future employers and service users of the professional's qualification. This is seen by most as a welcome development in increasingly complex work settings where clear standards must be maintained, and the risk of litigation is high if processes and quality standards are not enacted and met. However, it may be argued that an unintended consequence has been that the perceived value of informal learning, often work based, has been diminished. This is very concerning as a significant body of evidence across many fields suggests that work-based learning is a highly valuable component of any approach to CPD (Flanagan, Baldwin and Clarke, 2000).

Another consideration around the types of CPD you may seek to engage with are how you balance your specialist learning needs (e.g. CPD that specifically pertains to a technical component of your role, such as how a piece of specialist medical equipment is operated) and generalist needs (e.g. CPD that helps you to understand key changes to health and care in its broadest sense, such has how pharmaceutical medications and forms of treatment are assessed by the National Institute for Health and Care Excellence [NICE]). It could be argued that the general context in which you operate as a professional is equally as important as specialist knowledge and skills. However, the latter may seem more appealing when seeking to perform in a specific role, or differentiate your skill set in a competitive job market. Yet without an overview of the landscape in which you work it may not be possible to be a successful specialist practitioner in the longer term.

Healthcare professional regulators divide CPD into a range of different types. For example, HCPC differentiates between work-based learning, professional activity, formal education, self-directed learning and other types.

Work-based learning includes CPD activities such as learning by doing, case conferences, coaching from peers or senior colleagues, work shadowing, secondments, job rotation, journal clubs, supervising students or colleagues, visiting other departments (both within and beyond your employer) and reporting back, analysing watershed events, or undertaking a specific project.

As will be apparent from these noted work-based activities, these kinds of CPD can range from the relatively straightforward, such as taking the lead over selecting a journal article to discuss and critique with colleagues over a 30 minute session, through to the complex planning of a job rotation programme that may involve extended rotations either within or between health and social care employers.

When looking at a future or current employer it is important to analyse the breadth of work-based learning opportunities it offers to its employees.

Time for reflection

Think about the workplaces you have recently experienced. What evidence of work-based learning have you observed? Could more be done?

Developing a range of professional activities – such as lecturing or teaching, mentoring, giving a presentation as part of your employer's seminar series, becoming involved in a research project or becoming part of an internal or external working parties and groups – is a crucial part of the CPD mix. All of these activities will challenge you to think about your practice, consider the most contemporary evidence-based approaches and change your approach to work for the better. Moreover they will help to grow your internal and external profile and, if done well, will consequently increase your employability.

Formal education includes components such as university delivered courses, courses accredited by a professional body, attending scholarly conferences, writing articles or papers, or developing and delivering a course.

Self-directed learning is a very important component of CPD. Reading articles in peer reviewed journals in your areas of interest, specialist trade press (e.g. magazines, such as *Nursing Times*, or online publications from organisations, such as the BMJ) or organisations such as the Department of Health, Kings Fund, Healthwatch or the WHO should be a regular activity.

Similarly, it is worth exploring how you can use platforms such as YouTube, TED, Facebook, Twitter, LinkedIn, iTunes U, blogs, and Google Hangouts for your CPD. For instance, are you aware of all of the relevant experts in your field who Tweet? Do leaders in your field write a regular blog or have a YouTube channel? Are there groups on LinkedIn you can join? There is a massive variety of CPD-relevant content available on the Internet; the most challenging task is to keep on top of the most appropriate content for your learning needs.

Time for reflection
Think about your use of social media? How are you using it to support your CPD agenda?

Other broader civic activities, for example becoming a NHS Trust Governor, School Governor, Parish Councillor, or working for a charity may also be considered part of a meaningful CPD portfolio.

Ensuring that different types of CPD are recorded

At all times it is vital that you are collating evidence of your involvement and learning from CPD. In some cases, such as formal university courses with an examination, this is straightforward, as a certificate and grade are provided. However, where the learning is work based and more informal this can be more difficult, but common sense approaches are available.

For example, some CPD, such as case conferences, in-house seminars or reading peer reviewed journal articles, is unlikely to come with any form of certification. However, you can take sensible steps to document your attendance and learning from these events. For instance, case conferences or in-house seminars should have a sign-in sheet (if not create one, clearly capture the title, date and location of the event, ask all attendees to sign it, and ask the most senior person in attendance to sign it off as an accurate representation of those who attended). Scan or photocopy the sign-in sheet and distribute it to attendees so they can add it to their CPD portfolio. Secondly, it is advisable to allow, for example, 10 minutes at the end for attendees to work as a group to make some notes on a flipchart of the key learning from the session. Take a photograph of the flip chart paper using a digital camera on a mobile phone or tablet (obviously in some sessions during breakout groups some records of learning may well have already been captured – be sure to photograph these too). Then e-mail the photographs to attendees for their records. If they are used, also obtain (with the session leader's permission) a copy of any slides and hand outs (be very careful to anonymise any information that is confidential, such as patient identifiers).

When you are reading a journal paper, obtain a PDF copy, print it out, record the date you read the paper at the top, write notes directly on the paper highlighting your learning and then either keep it safely in a lever arch file, or scan a copy for your electronic portfolio. Alternatively, use one of the many PDF annotation software packages available (some of which can be freely downloaded) to directly write your notes on to the electronic version of the paper. From time-to-time it is important to cluster together journal papers you have read on related themes and bring together the learning, perhaps by identifying common themes in some reflective notes or a sketching out a mind map.

It is vital that you visit your regulatory body's web site to further consider the types of evidence it will accept as a record of your CPD.

Levels of CPD, credit-bearing or non-credit-bearing CPD

Important issues to address when thinking about your CPD mix is to consider the educational levels at which you have been learning, and whether or not the courses or programmes of study result in recognised awards.

Time for reflection

Is it essential that your CPD results in a recognised award, such as a Masters degree? Or can you evidence your CPD in other ways, such as creating a portfolio of your work-based learning?

Sometimes the level of intended learning is specified by CPD providers in terms of a job role (e.g. registered physiotherapist), by NHS Bands (e.g. suitable for Bands 5–7 occupational therapists) or by experience (e.g. suitable for registered practitioners in their first twelve months of practice).

A useful framework to consider the level of your learning is the Framework for Higher Education Qualifications in England, Wales and Northern Ireland (FHEQ). As shown in Table 4.1, the FHEQ summarises higher education qualifications into levels four to eight.

Table 4.1 Typical higher education qualifications for England Wales and Northern Ireland

FHEQ level	Typical higher education qualifications at each level
4	Higher National Certificate (NHC); Certificate of Higher Education (CertHE)
5	Foundation Degree (FdA, FdSc); Diploma of Higher Education (DipHE); Higher National Diploma (HND)
6	Bachelor's Degree with Honours (BA, BSc); Bachelor's Degree without Honours; Graduate Diploma; Graduate Certificate
7	Master's Degree (e.g. MA, MBA, MSc); Postgraduate Diploma (PgDip); Postgraduate Certificate (PgCert)
8	Doctoral Degrees (e.g. EdD, PhD/DPhil)

Registered health and social care professionals in the United Kingdom must now be educated to FHEQ Level 5 as a minimum, and most new entrants will be at Level 6 or higher.

If you have, for example, a Bachelor's Degree in Paramedic Science you will have completed 360 credits at Level 6. If then, for instance, you wanted to study an aspect of acute, critical or emergency care it is probably likely that you would seek to do so at Level 7 in order to further enhance your knowledge and skills level in your chosen fields. Perhaps you may elect to study a particular stand-alone credit-bearing module (e.g. 20 credits) at Level 7, or accumulate 60 credits (e.g. three 20-credit modules) to be awarded a PgCert, 120 credits (e.g. six 20-credit modules) to complete a PgDip or 180 credits (six 20-credit modules and, typically, a research project or service improvement project equivalent to 60 credits) to become recognised at the Master's Degree Level.

However, it may be the case that the same Paramedic Science graduate, when promoted to a management role, elects to study an unfamiliar topic (e.g. budget management) at Level 5 if that level provides the relevant learning outcomes. That said, it is equally acceptable for that graduate to engage with Level 7 study (e.g. a Masters of Business Administration [MBA]) on the basis that level of study will provide them with the learning outcomes they require and that they have successfully previously demonstrated the study skills and resilience to complete a Level 6 programme.

In summary, any learner engaging with credit-bearing CPD should consider the level at which they need to be able to apply the knowledge and skills in their current and anticipated future roles and the level of their own prior educational achievements specific to the country in which they wish to work.

One other point to bear in mind is that of the Accreditation of Prior Learning (APL) or Recognition of Other Learning (RoL). APL/RoL are mechanisms by which it may be possible to be awarded credits, at the appropriate FHEQ level, towards a university qualification (usually up to a maximum of 50% of the required credits) in other ways. For example, UK universities will generally consider the following categories of prior learning:

- Prior Certificated Learning, for example learning that is certificated and at a higher education level but has not led to the award of higher education credits, such as NHS 'in-house' training programmes.
- Prior Experiential Learning, for example relevant learning from vocational or other experiences which, when assessed by university academics, can lead to the award of university credits.
- Credit Transfer, for example where credits acquired at other UK higher education institutions can be transferred to a relevant programme of study at another UK university.

Where to access CPD

There are a broad array of providers, all of whom have strengths and potential weaknesses. The first port of call should be the workplace environment in which you are based. Can the CPD you need be arranged locally through a colleague who could act as tutor, mentor or coach? All high quality health and care providers should be dynamic training environments. For example, when a senior colleague carries out a particularly interesting procedure or comes across an interesting case, are colleagues invited, where appropriate, to observe the procedure as a learning opportunity or engage with the case?

Be sure to explore to see whether your employer has a virtual learning environment (VLE) where key learning resources are held. It is likely that the VLE will house key CPD-related documents, e-learning packages and other learning resources.

Your employer's intranet pages should set out in-house training opportunities and your employer's CPD lead or an appropriate HR manager with responsibility for workforce development should be able to provide further information.

Publishers of journals and trade papers often provide free or low cost CPD in areas related to their subject matter. The CPD is often written by experts and can be accessed at any time via e-learning. They may also convene CPD events such as regional study days.

Similarly, health-related charities and patient advocacy groups may provide various forms of face-to-face and e-learning in their areas of interest. Additionally, policy-related organisations, such as The King's Fund, often provide leading-edge CPD.

Learned societies focused on different specialist areas often convene CPD events, including study days and conferences. It is very important that you identify the UK-based and international learned societies in your areas of interest and look out for events such as webinars or Twitter chats.

Pharmaceutical companies and equipment manufacturers frequently offer very high quality CPD programmes in areas pertaining to their products and services. Most operate within clear ethical frameworks to ensure that the information they present is evidence based, objective and balanced. However, learners still need to be aware that one of the reasons why companies provide CPD is to try to increase the interest in, and the sales of, their products and services.

Universities are major providers of CPD and face-to-face learning can be undertaken at a local university. However, with the emergence of high quality e-learning it is now possible to register for courses of CPD study with universities across the globe. These international CPD events can be powerful ways to challenge your own views and approaches, and seek out new approaches to your work.

How to access CPD: Overcoming barriers

In a perfect world every health and care professional would have unlimited time and funding to access high quality CPD and apply their learning to practice. However, in the real world busy professional's work, family and free time is increasingly under pressure as life is lived at an increasingly fast pace. It is frequently cited in the literature that health and care professionals are being afforded insufficient time by their employers to undertake meaningful CPD, and the demands on their time away from work are increasing with respect to issues such as child care or looking after aging relatives, meaning that time to undertake CPD away from work is also limited (Joyce and Cowman, 2007). This means that professionals must work collaboratively with their employer to identify CPD that will deliver the greatest return on investment for the time spent learning.

A simple example may be to identify a CPD webinar that could be attended whilst at work, rather than having to commute to a venue. Or could you learn a technique through a series of observations of a senior colleague rather than attending a formal course? At a more sophisticated level, with reference to formal learning, can you consider whether the educational design of the course is likely to support the transfer of learning to practice?

Time for reflection

Consider how the recent learning you have undertaken could have been re-designed to become more time efficient.

One constant challenge is how to fund your CPD requirements. Fortunately, most employers have protected funds to support CPD. You will need to find out who controls these funds in your work environment. It is likely, for example, that if you work for the NHS there will be CPD lead for your locality and also for the wider Trust. If you look at the Trust intranet you should be able to identify how CPD budget is allocated in your workplace environment.

Frequently, companies, healthcare charities and patient interest groups offer CPD that is free of charge or heavily subsidised. Beyond that look for other sources of funding that may be available; these might include bursaries from professional bodies, trade unions, university alumni associations and local charitable organisations in your area, such as groups that support the local hospital (e.g. A League of Friends), or perhaps community organisations, such as the Rotary Club or Round Table. Crowd sourcing platforms may also be an option; for example, groups of healthcare professionals could launch a campaign to fund CPD in an area of particular interest to the general public.

Do make sure you explore all the free-of-charge options that may be available. There is now a huge selection of CPD provided by professional bodies, publishers and massive open online courses (MOOC) platforms (e.g. FutureLearn and Coursera). Important organisations, such as the Health Foundation and E-learning for Health, provide various forms of learning resources free of charge.

Obviously, self-funding of CPD can be an option, and at certain stages of your career it may be sensible (if you can afford to do so) to pay yourself for a course. For example, if you want to use the learning from the course to enable you to leave your current employer you will have a clear conscience when you come to hand in your notice. Also, on some occasions employers may say, for example, that if they fund your course you will have to pay back the course fees if you leave within a set period of time after completing the course. It is always worth checking to make sure that there are no written or implied terms associated with your employer funding a course.

Lastly, it should be mentioned that many healthcare professionals become frustrated when it appears that CPD opportunities may not be made fairly and equitably accessible to all grades of staff, and to all levels of experience. You need to understand the basis on which your employer makes CPD accessible to its staff. Is it based, for example, on identified need during appraisal or perhaps when senior management identify the vital areas in which CPD should be developed? You may need to make a strong case to justify your involvement in CPD. Do not simply walk into your line manager's office and ask to go on a course or for a secondment. It will be too easy for them to say no. Instead, link the CPD event to your last appraisal and your development needs, your performance objectives or a current project and how the CPD event will support the project. Provide them with an overview of the CPD event, its costs and the time it will take you away from your role. Most significantly, capture precisely how you think the CPD will change your practice, and how your learning will also support the development of colleagues.

Time for reflection

Consider some CPD you would like to engage with. How would you build the case to support your attendance at the event?

Evaluating the effectiveness of CPD

It is inevitable that some types of CPD will be more effective than others. However, given that we all have limited time and money to invest in CPD we have to work smartly to ensure that the CPD with which we engage is worthwhile.

It is obviously difficult to know in advance how valuable a CPD course or programme will be but, as mentioned elsewhere in this chapter, careful planning around whether, for example, it will meet your needs in terms of knowledge or skills deficits you are aware of, or if you will have the opportunity in your job role to deploy your learning, are imperative. Furthermore, where possible you should ask the provider of the CPD for feedback and case studies from participants on the course or programme and the employers of the participants. Obviously, in reality, most providers will showcase only the positive feedback, so where possible you should ask to speak directly to previous participants and their line managers.

Whether you speak to previous participants or have to rely on case studies or sound bites, there are frameworks that can help us dissect how valuable a given programme of work-relevant learning may be. For example, The Kirkpatrick Training Evaluation Model (Kirkpatrick, 1998; Kirkpatrick and Kirkpatrick, 1994) suggests that learning can be divided into four levels

- *Level 1: Reaction.* The first level in Kirkpatrick's model is called 'Reaction' and relates to whether students found the learning relevant to their needs and if they enjoyed the learning. This is normally assessed by a feedback sheet at the close of the learning event.
- *Level 2: Learning.* The second level is called 'Learning' and considers how students have learnt and retained the knowledge, skills and attitudes covered by the CPD. This level is assessed properly with a pre- and post-course test, such as a written examination or an OSCE.
- *Level 3: Behaviour.* The third level is called 'Behaviour' and is concerned with whether the accumulated knowledge and skills are deployed during day-to-day workplace activities, that is whether or not practice was changed as a consequence of the CPD. This element may require interaction with the student's line manager and colleagues, perhaps through feedback during an appraisal or a 360° feedback exercise, to explore how the student's approach and performance have changed and developed and whether this is directly linked to the CPD.
- *Level 4: Results.* Finally, level four is called 'Results' and considers if the CPD has ultimately had an impact on key deliverables. For example, in healthcare settings these may include target measures such as increasing patient satisfaction scores, reducing levels of recorded post-operative pain, reducing so called 'never events', or increasing the use of cheaper (but equally effective) medical equipment. The 'Results' level can be challenging to measure, as these impacts may take time (often months or years) to filter through to the workplace and determining whether or not the CPD was a causal factor for the change can be difficult to measure.

Kirkpatrick's model suggests that for work-relevant CPD to be deemed effective it should have a positive impact on each of the four levels. Therefore, when you see feedback from previous students you should carefully analyse what they say. For example, student A might have said 'The course was fantastic, I had a great time and learnt a lot about new approaches to dementia care. I would recommend it' while student B said 'The course was challenging in a good way, I was quickly able to learn new ideas and change my approach to working with service users living with dementia – and the feedback from service users' carers was fantastic'. Student A is perhaps reflecting that the CPD course s/he went on was effective for them at Kirkpatrick levels one and two, whereas Student B is implying that for them the learning was effective at levels one, two and three.

Time for reflection

Consider a recent learning activity you have undertaken. On which of Kirkpatrick's levels would you consider it to be effective and why?

An outline practical approach to planning and undertaking a balanced CPD portfolio

Any meaningful approach to CPD, irrespective of your clinical discipline, is underpinned by adhering to a set of key principles:

- *Recording*: Being meticulous in the way in which you keep a record of both your formal and informal learning.
- *Reflecting*: The act of capturing your thoughts in writing, or via a voice recorder, can support your learning and help you consider how you are transferring the learning to practice.
- *Tracking*: Look back every few months and consider what types of learning you have engaged with. Is it all formal or informal or is there a balance? Is it all specialist or generalist, or is there a balance? Is one project or CPD course dominating your efforts? Are you only engaging with topics you are comfortable with, or are you pushing out into new areas? Is your recording of CPD helping you to learn and document your learning, or is it inadequate? What is missing from your CPD mix?
- *Planning*: Once you have worked out what is missing from your CPD mix you need to plan how to respond to the identified gaps. Are you using your workplace appraisal to consider your performance and how CPD to improve it? Are you seeking feedback from colleagues to gain insight on your CPD needs? Are you thinking sufficiently about your career development plans and how this may impact your CPD agenda?
- *Reviewing*: Through the process of Recording, Reflecting, Tracking and Planning, you should be able to set out a clear examples of forward-looking CPD objectives. These objectives should be reviewed regularly by yourself, your line manager, mentors and other interested parties.

In terms of further building firm foundations to your approach to CPD, it is important to start out by really contemplating where you are in terms of your own development. It is often helpful to look at your current job specification, or if you are a student to look at role specifications for the types of jobs you would like to secure upon graduation. You may also want to reflect on your own CV and any recent reviews, such as your last performance appraisal, meeting with a mentor or a tutor. Consider four interrelated areas:

1. *Job-specific skills and knowledge*: The specific knowledge, skills and attitudes you have now that pertain to the job role you have *now* or aspire to acquire, and the *gaps* you perceive you have.

2. *Capabilities*: These are more generic competencies you may need in the workplace. For example the ability to be calm under pressure, lead new projects, manage a budget or listen to constructive feedback. Which key capabilities do you possess and which are you lacking? Also consider which of these competencies may be transferable into other roles or work settings

3. *Work values*: Give some thought to your values and what gives you satisfaction in your work. For example, are you driven by the challenge of being the best, leading the implementation of new approaches to work, acting as an advocate for service users, being the person in a team on whom others depend or feeling secure in your role. What drives you and leads to job satisfaction?

4. *Interests*: Also consider areas of life, both at work and beyond, that you find stimulating and rewarding. For example, do you enjoy organising events, reading, supporting others to bring the best out of them, being competitive and reaching targets, or helping people to learn?

From this described approach it can then be easier to sketch out an outline plan for the future. Clearly this plan may change, but writing down some aspirations can be helpful. For example:

- In 100 words or less think about where you aspire to be in two, five and ten years' time.
- In 100 words or less capture the strengths that will help you to achieve your stated aspirations.
- In a further 100 words consider the areas that require development which unless attended to will hold you back.

This will then enable you to start to set some clear CPD objectives that you can begin to develop and refine. From this, an action plan should start to emerge.

Conclusions

In summary, this chapter strives to get you thinking about your understanding of the role of CPD and its link to your current and future employability. CPD plays a significant role in ensuring that you provide safe and effective care to your patients, meet the demands of your employers, and develop a career that is rewarding. The learning in this chapter should enable you to think about how you plan, design, learn and apply your CPD to your job role.

Potential interview questions in this area
- Outline, with possible examples, the CPD you would like to undertake over the next 12 months. Why, in your view, will these lead to improved patient care?
- How have you identified in which areas you require CPD?
- Have you developed a CPD plan?
- How would you ensure that the learning from CPD is transferred into your practice?
- Are you aware of the different types of CPD your regulatory body require you to undertake?

References

Archer W and Davison J (2008) *Graduate employability: The views of the employers.* London: the Council for Industry and Higher Education (CIHE).

Blume B, Ford JK, Baldwin T and Huang J (2010) Transfer of training: A meta-analytic review. *Journal of Management,* **36**:1065–1105.

Flanagan J, Baldwin S and Clarke D (2000) Work-based learning as a means of developing and assessing nursing competence. *Journal of Clinical Nursing,* **9**:360–386.

Joyce P and Cowman S (2007) Continuing professional development: Investment or expectation? *Journal of Nurse Management,* **15**:626–633.

Kirkpatrick DL (1998) *Evaluating training programs: The four levels,* 2nd edn. San Francisco, CA: Berrett-Koehler Publishers.

Kirkpatrick DL and Kirkpatrick, JD (1994) *Evaluating training programs.* Berrett-Koehler Publishers.

Further reading

Brekelmans G, Poell RF and Van Wijk K (2013) Factors influencing continuing professional development: A Delphi study among nursing experts. *European Journal of Training and Development,* **37**:313–325.

Covell CL (2009) Outcomes achieved from organizational investment in nursing continuing professional development. *Journal of Nursing Administration,* **39**:438–443.

Gibbs V (2011) An investigation into the challenges facing the future provision of continuing professional development for allied health professionals in a changing healthcare environment. *Radiography,* **17**:152–157.

Haywood H, Pain H, Ryan S and Adams J (2012) Engagement with continuing professional development: Development of a service model. *Journal of Allied Health,* **41**:83–89.

Chapter 5 Leadership

Neil Sellen

Health Education East of England, Fulbourn, Cambridge, UK

Introduction

This chapter highlights the importance of developing leadership skills alongside your professional skills from the beginning of your career. It describes what we mean by leadership, how it applies in healthcare settings and what role leaders play. It considers the behaviours consistent with good leadership and asks you to consider the leadership style that fits your values and beliefs.

What is leadership?

Leaders inspire and encourage people to take on a goal or series of tasks that are beyond the individual alone. Leadership can be described as the use of particular behaviours that promote engagement, desire to achieve, collaboration, goal setting, delegation of tasks and celebration of achievements. All together, they help create a sense of team work, loyalty and common purpose, which makes achievement of objectives more possible than single enterprise. Leading others is, therefore, relationship based, as well as situational and related to position.

When we *talk* of leadership we often describe the actions and behaviours used to bring teams or individuals together to work on common goals. Leadership shows itself in many ways; it is affected by the task, the situation, the organisational, professional or team culture and by the psychology of the individuals involved. Leading is also informed and developed by followers; individually and collectively.

When we *think* of leadership, we often picture people who display the characteristics and behaviours we admire or dislike; or we associate the term with

How to Develop Your Healthcare Career: A Guide to Employability and Professional Development, First Edition. Edited by Lisa Taylor.
© 2016 John Wiley & Sons, Ltd. Published 2016 by John Wiley & Sons, Ltd.

feelings, an emotional reaction that arises from our personal experiences of leading or following. Leadership is also, therefore, a concept that can be either embodied or remain an aspiration.

Leadership can be displayed overtly, for instance in decision making and 'taking charge', or subtly, by creating the conditions in which others can thrive and achieve a goal. Leadership behaviours are not confined to the workplace, sports field or politics; they are employed daily as we chart our course through life. Whilst some consider leadership skills to be innate ('s/he is a born leader'), leadership behaviours can be learned, practiced and improved.

There are many different theories about leadership and different types of leading styles and behaviours. This chapter does not explore these theories but a series of recommendations for follow-up study are made at the end of the chapter.

Why is leadership important in health care?

Leadership is critical to the successful delivery of quality health care, which is delivered most effectively by teams of people. Each person has a specific role or expertise and it is the task of the leader to ensure that all team members can make their contribution and support each other for the benefit of the patient. What makes leading in healthcare different is that the team skills required to deliver good treatment and care can vary from one patient to another. This means that people move in and out of professional leadership situations as dictated by the needs of the patient. All this happens within the construct of a team or unit of people who also need support, leadership and management to help them do their jobs to the best of their abilities. Evidence shows that there is a strong correlation between the quality of leadership, the experience and productivity of individual team members and the quality of patient outcomes (West and Dawson, 2012).

That is, there is a direct link between an organisation with deficient leadership and, for example, higher than average mortality rates. The factor most closely associated with this outcome is that of organisational culture. Organisational culture is shaped by the decisions, actions and inactions of leaders. Put simply, good leaders can create cultures that support good care and safe practice (Schneider and Barbera, 2014).

The recent publication of reports into healthcare quality in the United Kingdom has highlighted the role and impact of leadership in the NHS in their findings (Francis, 2010, 2013; Berwick, 2013). Many of their findings around leadership are replicated in reports into social care, law enforcement and education as well as in health. These reports suggest that in health care, clinicians are insufficiently represented in general leadership positions.

Clinical leadership is being encouraged in both the NHS and private healthcare organisations, as evidence of the relationship between good clinical leaders and good healthcare quality is being established through research.

Leadership as a professional responsibility

All registered healthcare professions are regulated by a governing body, which sets and maintains the standards expected of professionals. Your regulatory body will have published information, direction or guidance for you, setting out its expectations of your professional responsibility around leadership. Each professional body will also have expectations regarding competency in leadership and standards of behaviour as a leaders and managers.

As a newly qualified healthcare professional, you will usually work in teams to deliver health care. You will be asked to contribute specialist knowledge and specialist leadership as you develop your career. You will also contribute to team and organisational culture, be asked to follow others at times and work as an equal member of a high performing team. It is essential that you take opportunities to develop your own leadership skills and experience as part of your continuing professional development and that you do so in accordance with your professional regulator.

Why choose to be a leader?

Improving care

Above all else, healthcare professionals should be focusing on the quality and safety of the treatment and care provided to their patients. Leaders can improve care well beyond their personal control but many do not *choose* to become leaders, they simply *become* leaders.

As a newly qualified healthcare professional you might see a better way for things to be organised in your workplace. Or you might want to introduce innovative practice to an established system – such as a service improvement idea, as discussed in the next chapter of this book. You will certainly be expected to work with others to deliver high quality, safe, professional care to patients. And you may see something about the way that the team works which could be improved.

The skills and behaviours needed to bring a team together and to change things are those which leaders use. In order to practice your professional skills to their fullest extent, you will need to develop your ability to lead. Good leaders are skilled in influencing thought, direction, policy and actions.

Influencing change

You may wish to share your research or clinical vision, or opinions and experience with others in order to promote your ideas more widely. Once again, the key leadership skills of building rapport, communicating a vision clearly and encouraging others are all essential to the spread of new ideas, techniques or behaviours. If you want to make a difference well beyond your own sphere of control you will need to influence others and shine a light for them to follow.

Reward and recognition

Reward and recognition in health care is usually related to your overall contribution to achieving the aims and objectives of your employer. This contribution can be affected by qualification, grade, level of specialism, level of professional responsibility, responsibility for resources and leadership. As you progress throughout your career you will often be given the opportunity to acquire additional responsibilities and be rewarded accordingly. The extent to which you exercise your leadership skills will, therefore, influence your career progression, earnings and recognition amongst your peers.

Because you have something to give

The modern healthcare sector is no longer a place where leadership is unquestionably hierarchical and inherent to a position. Leading today is personal, emotional, organic and fluid. It is not about power or status but about conviction, values and ethical behaviour. Today, a good medical/ surgical team will no long unquestioningly follow the lead consultant; it will question, challenge, contribute to decisions, review progress and develop as a team of equals. Your role as a newly qualified healthcare professional will be to share what you know, to learn more and to be a full and active member of your team. And if the occasion arises when you are called upon to lead in the interests of patient care and safety, you should feel ready to do so.

Case study

Four years after qualifying, Narinder was promoted to team leader. She now had newly qualified staff to deal with, as well as recruitment, covering vacancies and 101 other things that came with the role. Some of the other staff were a bit old fashioned in their practice and set in their ways. It was hard to make the changes she wanted, to sort out staff issues and still make time for direct patient care. Still, she learned quickly, loved her job and did her best. She made sure she took any professional development available and kept up her portfolio.

In time, Narinder was chosen to do some specialist training. She now had to work across several wards and did not get to spend so much time with the teams any more. When she did, it was to instruct them in procedures and lead her area of patient care. She liked the chance to make a difference but found some of the 'people stuff' a bit stressful. Why wouldn't people just get on with it? And why did they treat her differently now?

When she was offered some leadership development, Narinder was reluctant. She was not a leader, she was a specialist. But she knew she needed help, so she went for it.

During the programme, Narinder came to see that she was already a leader. Even if she did not feel like one, that is how others saw her. They looked to her for help to do their jobs better and they looked to her to sort out complex situations.

She realised that what she did influenced other people's behaviour and that they looked to her not just for professional guidance but for support and leadership. She started to practice some techniques that helped her manage herself better, be conscious of the impact she had on others and really understand what was behind some of the issues that kept coming up at work. This made her feel more confident in her ability to build relationships and be the leader people wanted her to be. With practice these skills helped her do her job better. She now felt confident that she could help others fulfil their own potential to improve care for patients.

She felt ready for the next big step....

Leadership and management

Most organisations need to establish a system of responsibility and accountability in order to be clear about the relationship between an individual or a team's role and the aims of the organisation as a whole. They define who is responsible for what. So we talk about people being responsible for managing budgets, managing people, managing equipment and managing tasks, and so on. Managers may be responsible and accountable for their area of control but they are not necessarily and automatically leaders. Some of the key differences in leadership and management are expressed by Northouse (2012), implying that leadership produces change and movement whereas management produces order and consistency. There are a number of examples of behaviours that would be consistent with leadership, such as establishing direction, as compared to management behaviour, such a planning and budgeting. In real life there are few roles where people will not be called upon to exercise skills from both of these paradigms. Managers will have explicit leadership roles and good ones will display behaviours that empower and enthuse people. They will also have to account for expenditure, carry out performance appraisals and react quickly to situations as they arise. Whilst leadership commentators like to play up the differences in approach, the reality is not so clearly defined. Leaders are expected to manage well and managers to lead.

Critically, for the newly qualified healthcare professional, there is not really an 'either/or' option with regard to management and leadership. As you increase your professional skills, you will be expected to take on greater management responsibilities. And as your management role expands you will be seen as a leader by others. It is important, therefore, to accept the need to develop the skills and behaviours of leaders and managers as integral to your continuous professional development throughout your career.

Leadership and culture

Organisational culture has a significant impact upon the success of the enterprise in achieving its goals. In NHS healthcare settings there appears to be a correlation between the culture, as expressed by staff satisfaction, and mortality. The research carried out by Michael West (2014) has suggested that leadership is the most important influence on culture:

> 'Every interaction by every leader in health care shapes the culture of their organisations. The best leaders promote partnership and parti-cipation and involvement as their core strategy; promote appropriate staff autonomy and accountability for improvement; ensure staff voices are encouraged encourage staff to be proactive and innovative...'

Good leaders West suggests '...avoid command and control except in crisis; take action to address system problems and unnecessary tasks that prevent staff from delivering high quality care'.

Above all, he continues, good leaders 'model compassion in dealing with patients and staff'.

In summary, it is a key task of all leaders to ensure that the culture of the organisation is supportive of the aims of that organisation. If it is not, it is their responsibility to challenge it and change it.

What is your approach to leading?

The following are all examples of effective leadership:
• Leading others to achieve goals.
• Leading thinking by sharing ideas.

- Sharing knowledge.
- Leading by example to establish standards.
- Commanding and controlling resource and task allocation.
- Lighting the way for others.
- Purposefully building collaborations, coalitions and networks to achieve an agreed, shared aim.
- Behaving in a way which aligns your actions with the values you espouse.

All have an appropriate place in every healthcare setting, every time an interaction takes place. The job of the healthcare worker is to adjust their approach to the setting and the occasion. In an emergency, you may need to take command of the situation and direct others. As a professional you may be asked to provide authoritative advice that will guide others' actions. As a mentor of others, you may be asked to guide self-reflection and self-development.

Time for reflection

Think now about your experiences of leadership in others and yourself:
- Who do you admire as a leader? Why?
- Is anybody you know a natural leader?
- What elements of what they do would you like to emulate?
- What model of leadership do you feel most comfortable with?

What do employers want in early and developing leaders?

Employers do not expect newly qualified professionals to display exemplary leadership behaviours from the beginning. These are honed over time and often not required in first roles. However, they will want to see evidence that the underlying personal values and qualities are in place. They will test these through interview, life history and, when in role, appraisal and development opportunities. Employability rests on your ability to demonstrate these personal qualities, above all self-awareness, alongside your professional skills and potential for development.

Most good employers will offer you the opportunity to discuss your development needs, usually annually. This is often called a 'development review' and is usually linked to a discussion about your performance at work. Doing some preparation before this review is an extremely good habit to form. Think about what you have done well at work, what you would like to improve on in the next 12 months. Crucially, think also about what skills you might need in your next role; start to prepare for it now by seeking to develop those skills before you need to rely on them.

What are the component behaviours and personal qualities that influence leadership effectiveness?

Having an understanding of what people may be looking for is an essential component of 'employability'. This enables you to consider how you can demonstrate 'fit' between your personal qualities and work or life experience and what the organisation wants. It also helps you to tailor your personal and professional development as you develop your career.

Component leadership behaviours

In their model, Holti and Storey (2013) identify nine component areas that they believe contribute to good leadership in healthcare settings. First among them is the ability to inspire shared purpose. Other components relate to the ability to manage oneself, to manage others and resources, to develop and promote a vision for improvement of health services and to make that vision a reality. It is important to note that every component in Holti and Storey's model is expressed in terms of the impact of behaviours and actions, not about beliefs and attitudes. This model suggests that it is what you do which is the most important part of leadership (how others experience you). The merit of this approach is that it suggests that you can change what you do, even if you find it harder to change how you feel. In this model, leadership can be practiced and if you are strong in one or more areas you can focus your development in other component areas. This model lends itself to 'stages' of development: from 'developing' to 'competent', through to 'excellence'. In this way, a common framework of behaviours can be built on throughout the course of your career.

Personal qualities

Personal qualities, such as self-awareness and self-management, are the bedrock for leading others. Important as they are, they are not the whole story. The additional component concerns the ability to relate to others, to empathise, to understand what motivates and to consider others' perspectives on issues and situations. Described variously as emotional intelligence, EI or EQ, this component is about how you connect to others in authentic relationships. Actions and behaviours that do not resonate with your true self can result in negative impact on your personal wellbeing and affect your relationship building with others (Kernis and Goldman, 2006).

What sort of leader are you?

Time for reflection

Thinking about you, now, what would you consider to be your natural leadership style? Think about an occasion when you have been called upon to show leadership:

- What was the situation?
- What did you do?
- What was the outcome?
- How did others react to you?
- How did you feel?
- What was the easiest part for you?
- What was the hardest?
- What would you like to have done differently?

You can assess your leadership capabilities through a series of assessment tools, which your employer may use during leadership development exercises. Some of the most commonly used tests are:

- *MBTI* (or, Myers-Briggs Type Indication): How we perceive the world and make decisions (http://www.myersbriggs.org/my-mbti-personality-type/mbti-basics/).
- *Belbin*: Describing the sorts of roles we prefer to play in a team (http://www.bclbin.com/).
- *Firo-B*: Considers how we relate to one another. How we want others to behave and how we tend to behave towards others (https://www.cpp.com/products/firo-b/index.aspx).
- *SJT* (or, Situational Judgement Test): For doctors in training. Describes a series of complex scenarios which a doctor may come across. The test considers situational judgement, or how one came to a decision (http://sjt.foundationprogramme.nhs.uk/).
- *360° Assessments*: Self, peer and manager assessment of the extent to which we behave in ways which conform to a paradigm of leadership. The object being to receive feedback from others on how the individual is perceived and compare it to their perception of self.

The purpose of each of these tools is to help answer the question: 'What is it like being on the receiving end of me?' They give you a sense of how you tend to approach situations and other people now. They describe the benefits and pitfalls of these styles or behaviours. Equipped with this self-knowledge and an insight into how your colleagues work, you will be able to think about your development needs as an individual, a team member and as a leader.

Typical leadership development activities

Many employers will offer a range of activities, programmes or workshops to help people with their development. Specialist providers may also be used. Activities range from access to assessment tools, an introduction to leadership, through to leadership qualifications. Typically, your journey will begin with:

- self-management
- assertiveness training
- managing difficult conversations
- leading a team
- leading change.

As your skills develop, you will build on these foundations and acquire new skills that help extend your influence and impact:

- coaching others
- influencing others
- leading teams
- leading services
- system leadership
- strategic leadership.

Employers' expectations of early career healthcare professionals

Employers will want to consider your potential for development throughout your career. They will usually want to explore areas such as personal initiative and interpersonal skills, which are the foundations of future leadership development. Above all else, they will want to know that your values will contribute to excellent healthcare provision.

You may be asked at interview to describe a situation from your personal life where you have taken a leading role. Or you may be asked how you would approach a situation which they describe. These questions are designed to understand if you understand your own impact in leading and what lessons you have learned from them. Think about how you might approach these questions in advance.

Time for reflection

What experiences from your personal life might you draw from in order to show an employer what sort of leader you might become?

Some sample interview questions are listed at the end of this chapter. Your employer will not expect well rounded, appropriate leadership skills in your first years as a practitioner. They will be looking for your interest in your personal development, your insight into your own behaviours and their impact upon others; they will look for any motivation to lead and they will want to see your flexibility of approach in different settings and situations.

When will you feel like a leader?

As a healthcare professional, it is likely that in the work setting the first leadership behaviours you will emulate and be expected to model will be professional. Your professional or specialist leadership will be called upon and expected as a natural part of your day.

In addition to this, your particular profession or specialism may already have role models and norms of behaviour that you will be expected to adopt as part of professional cultural identity norms. While there is an implicit expectation that you will adopt these, bear in mind that you are being inducted into a culture that may have developed over decades. It may not be appropriate in the context of modern health care and society's expectations. It is your professional responsibility to be accountable for your decisions and your actions and you should beware of conforming to established norms where they conflict with your personal values and the aims of high quality, safe patient care. You are a fresh pair of eyes, educated to a high standard and you should never be afraid to ask why things are done in a particular way. It may well be that there is no good reason to continue with outdated practice and your challenge will benefit the team as well as the patient.

As your career develops, your next leadership challenge is likely to be around the management of others (team leadership) or resources (money, equipment etc.). You will probably be expected to compete for roles where this is an adjunct to your professional career development. In one sense, therefore, the decision about whether you are ready for such responsibilities is shared between you and your employer. However, you will make your own judgement about your suitability and readiness for such roles. All good employers will assess your potential for success in role and be prepared to offer support for the development of skills and experience and to help you with the transition.

The essence of employability is to remain flexible. Being open to consider or reconsider the extent of your aspirations around leadership will mean that, when the time comes, you are in a position to take advantage of the opportunity to take on a greater leadership role and make a successful transition from your professional foundation to a wider leadership role.

The development of leadership skills is a journey, rather than a destination; one that will take you most of your working life. You may feel like a leader now or never feel like one; the key test of leadership is not how you feel but how others feel about what you do. You cannot be a leader unless others follow you.

Tips and trips

You are called on to exercise whatever leadership skills you have, in whatever setting you are, for the express purpose of delivering high quality, effective and safe health care. Any impact upon your personal career and standing with your peers is subordinate to that goal. The tips and trips below are suggestions to help you think through how you will approach this aspect of your work:

- Do not pretend to a knowledge or skill you do not have yet.
- Do be authentic. Be yourself. Every other option is too hard to maintain in the long run.
- Do not take on too much, too early. Confidence is an attractive trait; overconfidence can lead others to mistrust.
- Do accept that you will make mistakes as you develop as a leader. Always learn from them and guard against repeating them.
- Do not become the sort of leader others want you to be.
- Do choose your own style, practice it and refine it.
- Do not call yourself a leader. Others are the judge of your leadership skills.
- Do lead with purpose, for a purpose.

Time for reflection

You in five years' time

To help you think about your development needs, consider how you would see your future career developing. Think about:

- Where you want to be in relation to leadership.
- What skills you think you will need when you are there.
- What skills you already have.

Bridging the gap:

- How are you going to acquire the skills you need?
- What is your priority now?
  - o What can wait one year?
  - o What can wait three years?

Potential interview questions in this area
- Have you ever had to bring others around to your way of thinking? How did you approach it and what happened?
- What has been your greatest challenge? Why? What did you learn about yourself? What would you do differently now?
- Describe a situation in which you have led. What happened? Why did it happen?

References

Berwick D (2013) *A promise to learn – a commitment to act: Improving the safety of patients in England.* Accessed at https://www.gov.uk/government/uploads/system/uploads/attachment_data/file/226703/Berwick_Report.pdf (last accessed 10 August 2015).

Francis R (2010) *Robert Francis Inquiry report into Mid-Staffordshire NHS Foundation Trust.* Accessed at http://webarchive.nationalarchives.gov.uk/20130107105354/http:/www.dh.gov.uk/en/Publicationsandstatistics/Publications/PublicationsPolicyAndGuidance/DH_113018 (last accessed 10 August 2015).

Francis R (2013) *Report of the Mid Staffordshire NHS Foundation Trust Public Enquiry.* Accessed at http://www.midstaffspublicinquiry.com/ (last accessed 10 August 2015).

Holti R and Storey J (2013) *Towards a new model of leadership.* Accessed at: http://www.leadershipacademy.nhs.uk/wp-content/uploads/2013/05/Towards-a-New-Model-of-Leadership-2013.pdf (last accessed 10 August 2015).

Kernis M and Goldman B (2006) A multicomponent conceptualization of authenticity: Theory and research. In MP Zanna (ed.), *Advances in experimental social psychology* (pp. 284–357). San Diego, CA: Elsevier Academic Press.

Northouse P (2012) *Leadership: Theory and practice*, 6th edn. London: Sage Publications.

Schneider B and Barbera K (eds) (2014). *Oxford handbook of organizational climate and culture.* New York: Oxford University Press.

West M (2014) The NHS needs a leadership revolution. *The Guardian*, 22 May [online]. http://www.theguardian.com/healthcare-network/2014/may/22/nhs-needs-leadership-revolution (last accessed 8 August 2015).

West M and Dawson J (2012) *Employee engagement and NHS performance.* Accessed at: www.kingsfund.org.uk/sites/files/kf/employee-engagement-nhs-performance-west-dawson-leadership-review2012-paper.pdf (last accessed 10 August 2015).

Further reading

Barr J and Dowding L (2012) *Leadership in healthcare*, 2nd edn. London: Sage Publications.

Hartley J, Martin J and Benington J (2008) *Leadership in healthcare – A review of the literature for healthcare professionals, managers and researchers.* Accessed at http://

www.nets.nihr.ac.uk/__data/assets/pdf_file/0003/64524/FR-08-1601-148.pdf (last accessed 10 August 2015).

NHS Leadership Academy (2013) *NHS healthcare leadership model.* Available at http://www.leadershipacademy.nhs.uk (last accessed 10 August 2015).

Northouse P (2015) *Leadership and practice.* London: Sage Publications.

West M, Eckert R, Steward K and Pasmore B (2014) *Developing collective leadership for healthcare.* The Kings Fund. Accessed at http://www.kingsfund.org.uk/sites/files/ kf/field/field_publication_file/developing-collective-leadership-kingsfund-may14.pdf (last accessed 10 August 2015).

Chapter 6 **Service improvement**

Jonathan Larner
School of Health Sciences, University of East Anglia, Norwich, UK

Background and context

In the previous chapter we looked at the importance of developing your leadership skills from the beginning of your career. In this chapter we are going to examine how service improvement experience can help you to develop both essential and desirable employability skills. During this chapter we will explore these skills so that you can recognise for yourself how your service improvement experience can help you to get the career or job you really want. As this is an area where your emerging leadership skills can be further developed and honed, we will come full circle at the end of the chapter by summarising how service improvement is integral to healthcare leadership.

As a healthcare professional there are many things that you can do to market yourself to potential employers. First and foremost, in order to secure work it is essential that you are able to demonstrate that your personal profile fits the specifications of the job description. In other words, you must be able to show that you are fit for purpose. However, in the current highly competitive job market it is likely that you will be part of a large pool of appropriately qualified healthcare professionals, all keen to demonstrate their potential value. With this in mind one, of the most useful pieces of advice I was given as a new graduate was to carefully consider what added value I could bring to potential employers. Whilst there will undoubtedly be many ways that you can show how you offer something unique, certain types of activity and experience lend themselves particularly well to this purpose. Service improvement is a great example of an area where knowledge and experience can provide you with a wealth of transferrable employability skills and, therefore, the opportunity to clearly demonstrate to employers how you will be an asset to the team in the future.

How to Develop Your Healthcare Career: A Guide to Employability and Professional Development, First Edition. Edited by Lisa Taylor.
© 2016 John Wiley & Sons, Ltd. Published 2016 by John Wiley & Sons, Ltd.

It is important to point out at this stage that a propensity for improvement and managing change is actually a fundamental requirement for modern healthcare professionals that will undoubtedly be written into all job specifications. Yet, despite this fact, relatively few healthcare graduates really grasp the value of fully engaging with service improvement. When you analyse the many transferrable skills that can be evidenced by demonstrable service improvement experience, even at a very basic level, hopefully you will begin to see that this is your opportunity to show potential employers how you can make a real difference to their organisation.

So is it feasible for students and new graduates to be realistically expected to be improvers when they are still coming to terms with the basics of service delivery? The answer to this is emphatically 'yes'. The reason for this is that service improvement methodology is logical and objective. It generally starts with a picture of what is happening currently, in order to help everyone to visualise where improvements need to be made. To do this does not require you to be an expert. Instead it requires you to be able to build up an accurate picture of what is currently happening by consulting widely with all of the stakeholders involved. One effective way of doing this is by using a simple tool such as a 'Process Map' (NHSI, 2007), which is essentially a flow chart of the work process that acts as a visual representation of what is actually happening in practice. As well as being beneficial for actually being able to picture all of the critical stages within the process, the act of producing the map requires you to discuss what is happening with team members. The finished process map then acts as evidence for the team to brainstorm to find ways of improving the service. In this way, the application of common sense and objectivity is just as valuable as experience. In fact, when it comes to thinking innovatively or creatively about how to do things differently, a fresh pair of eyes can be a distinct advantage (Adair, 2012).

Although a fresh pair of eyes is very valuable when looking for new ways of working, it is essential that everyone involved in the work process is consulted during the service improvement process. In fact, when analysing services it is absolutely vital that all of the team members are able to contribute, ideally in the same room at the same time. This will ensure that the outcome accurately reflects what is happening in reality and not just what certain people think is happening. Importantly, working through this mapping process together promotes a sense of collective ownership and involvement in the improvement; this will increase the chances that any proposed change will be successful. Indeed, it is through this process that ideas for improvement normally begin to flow and can be actively encouraged from all members of the team.

However, before we get too carried away, it is very important to recognise that analysing services and suggesting areas for improvement is the relatively simple part. Making sure that the improvements suggested are meaningful and can be implemented in practice is a much harder job. Ensuring that the improvements 'stick' in the long term, that is they are sustainable over time, is even harder. Much of this depends on the ability of the whole team to work together to collectively own the improvement and to methodically work through progressive cycles of change to iron out the many problems that present themselves in practice. Based on original work by Walter Shewhart, American change guru W. Edwards Deming developed a model to ensure that changes are carefully planned, implemented, monitored and maintained long term. His 'Plan, Do, Study, Act' (PDSA) cycle (also known as the Deming wheel) has been widely adopted within healthcare improvement as it is simple and logical to use (Langley *et al.*, 1996). However, Deming identified that even the most simple change is likely to require numerous PDSA cycles to be undertaken before the change becomes embedded in practice, with each subsequent cycle refining the process yet further.

Now let us go back to the interview situation and consider how an employer is likely to view someone who not only understands how to analyse work processes in order to find ways to improve, but is able to demonstrate understanding of the 'human factors' associated with behavioural change. Clearly this person is going to have a greater chance of convincing employers that they can make a difference in the tough world of work. Of course, no employer can realistically expect a new graduate to be an expert in this field. However, engaging with even simple improvement projects will provide you with considerable experience that will help you to start developing the resilience that is vital for seeing changes through from the drawing board to measurable, sustainable improvement in the real world. This chapter is intended to help you to see this for yourself and, therefore, to inspire you to learn more about service improvement and managing change.

Where has service improvement come from?

Improvement methodology is certainly not a new concept. Wherever there is a desire to make things better, there will be people working to find the best ways of doing it. In the business world there are always innovative people searching for new ideas or new products, and trying to find ways to produce them more cheaply. It is, therefore, not surprising that there have been a number of different quality improvement models used within the field of industry, particularly manufacturing, since the beginning of the twentieth century. The car industry is particularly renowned for innovation and improvement. This dates right back to the time that Henry Ford developed mass-production techniques for his new Model T, which allowed a car to be constructed in an incredible 93 minutes in 1911! Improvement methodology became more widely recognised and acknowledged in the 1950s when Toyota's Taichi Ohno founded the Toyota Production System. In the latter half of the last century, Japanese manufacturers were renowned for successfully producing innovatively designed cars that were superior, yet cheaper than their American competitors. In the 1980s America responded to this competition and it was around this time that the work of American quality systems expert W. E. Deming proved to be the stimulus for what we now know as the modern quality and process improvement movement (Hunt, 2010).

Service improvement methodology has really only been applied within the NHS in relatively recent times. Between 2006 and 2013, the NHS Institute for Innovation and Improvement (NHSI) developed initiatives such as the Productive Ward Series, to help NHS teams to redesign and streamline the way they manage their work. The aim of this initiative was to improve the quality of care by reducing unnecessary waste of resources, therefore freeing up more time to care. It used efficiency techniques previously developed within car manufacturing and the aviation safety industry, and adapted them for use in the NHS. This type of innovation has led to the promotion and development of a continuous improvement culture within the NHS over recent years.

Despite the relative infancy of service improvement methodology within the NHS, quality of care has been firmly on the agenda for a number of years. In 1998, the Department of Health (DoH) white paper '*The new NHS: modern, dependable*' first described clinical governance as 'a system for ensuring that clinical standards are met and that processes are in place for continuous improvement' (Scally and Donaldson, 1998). Subsequent to this publication the NHS spent the next ten years developing systems and processes to underpin clinical governance, with every healthcare professional made accountable for playing their part in delivering it. Yet, despite all of this effort, when Lord Darzi reviewed the NHS in 2008, he identified the need to make the NHS safer, more clinically effective and more personal. Looking forward ten years to the NHS of 2018, Lord Darzi indicated that the NHS is likely to be substantially different, with greater emphasis placed on prevention, individual empowerment, quality of care and integration of services. He stressed the need to 'unlock local innovation and improvement' and to 'empower frontline staff to lead change that improves quality of care for patients'. To make it really clear to everyone what people should expect of the new NHS, Darzi introduced the NHS Constitution. This document sets out the 'commitments to patients, public and staff in the form of rights to which they are entitled and pledges which the NHS will strive to deliver, together with responsibilities which the public, patients and staff owe to each other to ensure that the NHS operates fairly and effectively' (DoH, 2013a).

The drive for innovation and improvement over recent years has been supported by the introduction of the Quality, Innovation, Productivity and Prevention (QIPP) challenge (DoH, 2013b). QIPP is a resource for everyone working in the NHS, public health and social care for making decisions about patient care and the use of resources. It was designed to support the NHS to make efficiency savings that can be reinvested back into the service to continually improve quality of care. Andrew Lansley, who was the Secretary of State for Health at the time, emphasised the need for healthcare providers to do things differently:

> 'All those who work on the frontline should be thinking carefully, and imaginatively, about how we can do things differently. The QIPP process is a home for this in the NHS and the way that we can implement the best and brightest ideas across the service'.
> Andrew Lansley, Secretary of State for Health, 2010

The threat that has to be managed during this time of change is that drives for efficiency may compromise the quality and safety of the care provided. It has been in the midst of this emerging drive to think innovatively about service delivery that a number of high profile scandals have become apparent. The events that unfolded at the Mid-Staffordshire NHS Trust clearly illustrated how things can go very badly wrong within an organisation that is under pressure to become more efficient. The inquiry report by Francis into the events at Mid-Staffordshire (Francis, 2013) proved to be a watershed moment for the NHS, with around 280 recommendations proposed by the report. The catastrophic series of events that Francis highlighted illustrated how an organisation can lose track of the values laid out in the NHS Constitution and allow safety and quality to be dramatically compromised in a culture driven exclusively by achieving financial balance and reaching targets. Whilst the future sustainability of the NHS demands that we find ways to deliver health care more efficiently, simply cutting costs will not be the answer. Public sector consultant Rob Worth (2011, p. 7) advocates that service improvement is the best way to reduce costs, stating that 'good work costs less'. He stresses that cost cutting always leads to deterioration in the service, which, in turn, leads to higher costs when dealing with the many consequences of bad service. He explains that history clearly shows us that if we focus on improving the quality of services by designing processes that deliver value for the service user and get rid of waste wherever possible, this, in turn, delivers considerable cost savings.

Therefore, it is in the light of the Francis Inquiry Report (2013) that service improvement should be viewed. If we are to successfully redesign processes and working practices in order to both save money and improve quality, there has to be a formal way for staff to identify where improvements can be made and to manage the implementation of those changes. These improvements can be driven by the desire to improve the quality of care and by the desire to use resources as efficiently as possible. The two are not mutually exclusive. Service improvement methodology provides the tools that healthcare teams can use to find the right way forward under challenging circumstances.

How does service improvement feature in healthcare education?

Given the relatively recent introduction of service improvement methodology in the NHS, it is not surprising that it has not been part of the taught curriculum for healthcare students until recent years (NHSI, 2008). In his 2008 review of the NHS, Lord Darzi recognised the important role of the next generation of healthcare professionals in the design and delivery of healthcare services. He directed a new challenge for healthcare education to produce a workforce capable of achieving the significant challenges facing modern health care. More specifically, Darzi's '*A high quality workforce: NHS next stage review*' (Darzi, 2008) defines how the NHS, higher education and industry should work together to improve the skills and competencies of the work force with the ultimate aim of improving the quality of services offered in the NHS.

In 2006, the NHSI, working in conjunction with Warwick University, began developing a programme of service improvement training that it believed could be relatively easily embedded into the curriculum for all healthcare students (Lister, Larner and Lynch, 2011). It embarked upon a widespread programme of education for Higher Education Institutes (HEIs) across the country and invited any HEI that was delivering education to healthcare professionals of any discipline, to join the programme. By 2010 there were over 50 universities involved and the teaching had been rolled-out to an estimated 10 000 students across the United Kingdom (Lister, Larner and Lynch, 2011). At the University of East Anglia we have been an active partner in this process and have developed our own model of service improvement teaching that incorporates all of the key elements recommended by the NHSI (Larner, 2012a, Larner and Collier, 2012).

Our experience of setting students a real service improvement task to undertake during practice placements has been extremely positive. Not only have we found that students are able to use a process mapping tool to analyse an aspect of a clinical service, but that they are consistently able to identify and suggest improvement ideas that could be implemented in practice. The feedback received on these tasks from the practice educators who supervise the students has been overwhelmingly positive. The ultimate value of this service improvement teaching will be measured in the future, by identifying whether graduates have been able to use their newly developed knowledge and skills to implement meaningful and sustainable service improvements in practice. However, there are numerous immediate benefits of this teaching that have become evident to us as we have developed our service improvement teaching (Larner, 2012b). These relate to the very nature of service improvement and the behaviours and attitudes that underpin the methodology. It encourages you as a student to develop your creative thinking, to take an innovative and entrepreneurial approach, and to challenge many of the assumptions that underpin our everyday working. Students value the opportunity to communicate effectively with the whole multidisciplinary team and, ultimately, to work within teams to bring fresh perspectives to the workplace. If we look at employment more broadly for a moment, there is a strong correlation between these types of activity and what employers want from you as a graduate. For example, the Confederation of British Industry (CBI) states that graduates need to be able to demonstrate a positive attitude, a 'can-do' approach, a readiness to take part and contribute, openness to ideas and a drive to make things happen (Lowden et al., 2011).

The literature indicates that employers want graduates who can adapt to the workplace culture, use their abilities and skills to evolve the organisation and participate in innovative teamwork. Employers also value critical thinking and reflection, as these skills are required for innovation and anticipating and leading change (Harvey et al., 1997; Little, 2001, in Lees 2002). Each of these things can be ably demonstrated through engagement with service improvement. We have found that the majority of our students are able to use any experience, however small, to demonstrate how they would transfer these valuable skills to any potential new working environment. By doing this they are also able to show that they are innovative, creative and team-focused.

Service improvement as an 'employability skill'

Hillage and Pollard (1998) described employability as the knowledge, skills, attitudes and behaviours required by individuals to seek, obtain and sustain employability at all levels in the labour market. Some fairly comprehensive employability skills-mapping exercises have been carried out in the field of health care over recent years, in order to help both employers and staff to understand the requirements of different job roles at different levels. Two examples are particularly worthy of mention, as between them they cover a very wide range of generic employment roles and responsibilities across the whole health sector.

1. **The Knowledge and Skills Framework KSF for Health** (DoH, 2004; NHS Employers, 2010)
   A broad, generic framework designed to be widely used across the UK NHS. It identifies the core knowledge and skills that individuals need to be able to demonstrate when applying for employment, using a consistent language and common classification. The KSF was simplified and relaunched in 2010 after independent review by the NHS Staff Council.

2. **The Employability Skills Matrix ESM for the Health Sector** (Skills for Health, 2014)
   A practical tool developed by Skills for Health, the Sector Skills Council for all health employers, NHS, independent and third sector organisations. It identifies the typical personal skills, qualities, values, attributes and behaviours required for working in health care. Like the KSF, it is intended to support staff in their career development; but it is also a useful resource that assists employers and commissioners in defining the employability skills required by staff working at different career levels and in different roles across the wider healthcare sector.

Both of these mapping tools are useful to look at when you are preparing for a job interview because they put service improvement into context with the overall package of employability skills you will be expected to demonstrate in your new job role. Therefore, they will help you to put what you have learnt from your experience into words that relate to these expectations. Irrespective of where you work, both tools can be considered helpful for conceptualising how you have developed valuable transferrable skills in the language that employers understand and appreciate, which will enhance your chances of securing the job you want.

What level of service improvement experience will be expected?

The relative importance placed on having some experience of service improvement is clearly demonstrated within the Knowledge and Skills Framework by the fact that it is one of the six core dimensions identified. Four levels of experience are identified within the KSF, which should give you some idea about where your personal knowledge and skills fit.

Level 1

The most basic KSF level expects that employees are able to 'make changes to their own practice and offer suggestions for improving services'. It is worth noting that it is an expectation that any member of staff, whatever their role or responsibility, is able to do this. Therefore, an employer will expect you to be able to talk about it. You should start by asking yourself if you can recall times when you have made suggestions for improving a service and how you did this. What evidence do you have that your ideas were listened to and whether they were helpful and constructive? This highlights the value of keeping a track of all of the improvement ideas you have had, what has provoked them and what tools you may have used during the analysis of the problem. Here an employer is most likely going to be looking for enthusiasm and passion for improvement, with the emphasis being on ideas and suggestions rather than actual improvement projects. Some creative thinking, some basic awareness of service improvement tools and a willingness to get involved are, therefore, an advantage.

Level 2

This level expects that employees are able to 'contribute to the improvement of services'. Showing an awareness of how and why engagement is required at this level is essential for healthcare graduates. Although most students will have been taught some theory of service improvement somewhere in their educational programme, an employer will be looking for more here. Whilst all of the things highlighted in level one are still likely to be valuable, it is most likely that a lack of structure and logical thinking will find many people out at this level. Therefore, this is where you need to be able to call upon some real examples of service improvement activities that you have been involved with. They do not all have to be fantastic winning ideas that saved lots of money, although that would be nice! My advice here would be for you to identify some good examples of small improvement projects you have been involved with and analyse them carefully in advance. In case you are unclear of what types of experiences count as service improvement, some real life examples of student projects are given at the end of the chapter in the case studies section.

It is highly unlikely as a new graduate that you will have had the opportunity to take an idea right through from the problem to the solution. Therefore, you almost certainly will not have been able to follow the cycle further down the line to assess the impact. However, if you have been involved with two or three good ideas as a student, and you can understand the theory and reflect on the learning outcomes of your project, then you will be able to talk with some authority on how you can contribute to the improvement of services.

Level 3

At this level an individual is expected to 'appraise, interpret and apply suggestions, recommendations and directives to improve services'. Not all new healthcare graduates will be able to demonstrate actual engagement at this level, but some will. Here lies a clear opportunity for individuals to set

Time for reflection
- What was the problem and how did you go about analysing it?
- Who was involved and who did you talk to?
- What tools did you use?
- What was your improvement idea?
- What were the benefits of what you did?
- What were the barriers to change?
- How would you measure the impact of your idea in the future?
- How will you make sure your change is sustainable in the future?

themselves apart from the crowd by showing how they have engaged at this level by really applying theory to practice. Graduates who have undertaken practical service improvement tasks whilst on practice placement will have a distinct advantage here and evidence of implementing even basic improvements is likely to be received well by employers. Nevertheless, if you have not had the opportunity to do this during your training you do not need to panic. Graduates who can show that they appreciate how service improvement might be applied in practice should still be able to perform well at interview.

Level 4

This level expects employees to 'work in partnership with others to develop, take forward and evaluate direction, policies and strategies'. Normally this would not be an expectation of new healthcare graduates, being more the remit of experienced leaders and managers. Nevertheless, an awareness of these higher level expectations of service improvement would show leadership aspirations. There is a balance to be found here between confidence and arrogance when it comes to articulating one's own skills and knowledge, particularly when experience is limited. However, if well evidenced a discussion of this nature would be recognised by most employers as leadership potential.

What specific skills can I demonstrate through service improvement experience?

The Employability Skills Matrix (ESM) provides guidelines for how employees working in different jobs can be aligned to nine different functional levels of employment. This framework starts at level 1, which is initial entry level, and rises to level 9 for the most senior staff within an organisation. Each level has a descriptor which identifies the types of staff whose job roles will fit within that level. A healthcare graduate will typically start work at level 5 of the Career Framework, referred to as practitioner level. The aim of the ESM is to provide a common language to assist both staff and employers with the mapping of employment skills, allowing you to see how you are expected to progress with each subsequent career step. One of the benefits of the ESM is that it allows you to identify how transferable skills may be relevant to other job roles, including those that are not readily identified via traditional routes.

The ESM approaches employability skills in a different way to the KSF. Rather than identifying specific topics or dimensions, it highlights the personal skills, qualities, values, attributes and behaviours that are expected of people working at each of the nine levels of the Career Framework. Once again improvement (and numerous associated terms) features at every level, even at entry level. This once again highlights the importance of service improvement experience when you are aiming to demonstrate that you are the right person for the job.

There are numerous skills, qualities, values, attributes and behaviours identified under level 5 (Practitioner Level) that can convincingly be demonstrated through service improvement experience; the following have been selected as examples for you to consider (Skills for Health, 2014, p. 21).

Communication and customer care
- Listen to and ask a variety of questions to understand the points of view of others, including team members and service users.
- Persuade and influence others.
- Proactively raise concerns about the provision of services to service users with supervisor and managers.

Solving problems
- Assess situations and identify the root cause of a problem.
- Seek different points of view, including the views of service users, and evaluate them on the basis of facts.
- Readily use theoretical and practical knowledge to think, gain and share information, solve problems and make decisions.

All of these communication and problem-solving skills are required to successfully engage with service improvement methodology in practice. Identifying where problems exist and then exploring the processes or practices involved with all of the key stakeholders is a fundamental part of any improvement project. A constructive approach to finding the root cause of the problem can be ably demonstrated by the methodical use of improvement tools, and a proactive approach will be evident through your drive to find a solution to the problem. Your ability to effectively collect and present evidence that shows what the problem is and how it can best be addressed will be an excellent way to demonstrate that you are capable of evaluating things on the basis of facts. In addition, you can show your ability to persuade and influence by demonstrating how you have presented this evidence to others in support of your improvement idea.

Mathematics

- Evaluate equipment, techniques and procedures with the aim of improving efficiency and effectiveness.

For an improvement idea to be successfully implemented it is essential that there is a clear idea of how the impact of the change will be measured. Therefore, during any change cycle there will be a need to collect, analyse and present data to monitor and evaluate the improvement. Experience of service improvement is, therefore, very good for developing and demonstrating the mathematical skills required for working in a modern healthcare environment.

Working with others

- Work with others towards achieving shared goals to improve and maintain the quality of service provision.
- Respect and be open to the thoughts, opinions and contributions of others, including colleagues, and service users.
- Develop, with the team, a clear purpose and objectives to improve and maintain the quality of service provision.
- Proactively identify creative and transferable solutions in relation to specific problems or conflict.
- Provide leadership and/or support to others when appropriate, motivating a group to achieve high performance and cope with unpredictable change.

As service improvement is rarely undertaken alone, engagement with this type of activity will be very powerful for demonstrating effective team working. Working on a process map within a team, ensuring that everyone's views are included and represented, and bringing the whole team along with you as the improvement idea is proposed and implemented, requires a range of these transferrable skills. Even though you may not have been able to gain experience in actually implementing improvement ideas, an awareness of the impact of change on teams and the many barriers that present in practice, will be extremely valuable. If you can also provide some potential strategies for overcoming those barriers, you will demonstrate a propensity to provide leadership and support during a change process, which are highly desirable traits for employers.

Demonstrate positive attitudes, values and behaviours

- Identify and suggest alternative ways to get the job done whilst maintaining a compassionate and caring service provision.
- Be creative and innovative in implementing solutions, maintaining honesty, integrity and transparency.

- Make best use of resources including time, to achieve agreed goals for service delivery, taking responsibility for own actions and self-development and providing effective team leadership.
- View change as an opportunity and cope with uncertainty, assessing and minimising risk.

Perhaps one of the most powerful benefits of engaging with meaningful service improvement activity is that is shows you have a positive attitude towards improving quality. Talking with confidence about your real experiences of how you have worked with a team to identify an area for improvement will help convey your desire to take responsibility for making the best use of resources through looking for ways of doing this differently. This may well involve creative and innovative ideas for improvement and will certainly demonstrate that you are the type of person who will embrace change and be proactive in looking for opportunities to improve.

Service improvement and leadership skills

In 2011, NHS Chief Executive Sir David Nicholson recognised that during a time of significant change for health and care services there is a need for 'bold and thoughtful leadership, rethinking how we work, challenging current practice and thinking outside of our own organisation and professional interests (NHS Leadership Academy, 2011, p. 5).

If you have engaged in service improvement activities you will undoubtedly have demonstrated positive leadership skills. A person who engages with improvement activities will display the confidence to question the way things are done and a willingness to think creatively about changing practice. They will need diplomacy and sensitivity, as people often feel defensive when practice is being challenged. They will need to be able to encourage and motivate the whole team of people involved to work together in analysing their service to identify where things need to improve and then to find a meaningful solution. Once the need for improvement is established, leadership skills are required to bring together everyone's opinions and ideas about what to do about it. Although it will often be an individual who comes up with an improvement idea, the team must appreciate and understand this idea if it is going to be successfully implemented. Leadership skills are then required to motivate the team to change what they are doing currently and to ensure that the impact of the change is fully evaluated. Many ideas fail at this stage because the human factors associated with change have not been carefully considered. If you can indicate how you might be able to lead your team successfully through an improvement cycle and help them to address the challenges associated with a change process, you will indeed be exhibiting leadership potential that any employer would value.

Conclusions

The intention of this chapter has been to help you recognise the importance and value of service improvement experience. I have argued that the knowledge, skills, attitudes and behaviours that you develop when doing this type of work will be in high demand amongst modern healthcare employers, with service improvement experience potentially demonstrating all of the following:

- A caring and compassionate attitude towards others by trying to make services the best they can be for everyone involved.
- Logical and objective thinking to analyse the current service.
- Creativity and innovative thinking when making improvement suggestions.
- Collaborative team work to ensure everyone's voice is heard.
- A quality-driven approach to work consistent with the principles of clinical governance.
- A problem-solving approach to finding the best possible solution available.
- Change management skills through the development of strategies to overcome barriers and make improvements sustainable.
- A positive can-do attitude to doing things differently.
- Leadership skills in motivating and driving your team through change.

By systematically reflecting on your own personal experiences of service improvement and mapping them against tools such as the KSF and the ESM, you will be able to use evidence that you have at your disposal to articulate how you have developed some or all of these skills. This will help you to demonstrate how you are developing into a highly effective practitioner who is well positioned to impress in an interview situation.

Case studies

Three real life examples of student service improvement ideas are presented here. They have been selected as typical of the types of improvement ideas that University of East Anglia students come up with on a regular basis.

Case study 1
Name: Physiotherapy Student
Placement Type: Orthopaedic Hospital Ward

Background – This should include your aim (what you are trying to accomplish)

Give a description of the problem and your identification of the need for improvement including any implications for patients, carers and staff.

Problem: Total hip or knee replacement patients who were put on the 'enhanced recovery programme' (ERP) are frequently not discharged from hospital any quicker than those not put on the programme.

Need for improvement: One shortfall of the ERP is that a physiotherapist should see the patient on the same day as surgery (day 0). However, this is often impractical for three reasons:

1. The patient returns back to the ward late afternoon (the physiotherapist has finished for the day).
2. The recent anaesthetic makes mobilisation unsafe.
3. The patient is drowsy, which can limit exercise concentration and compliance.

If a post-operative patient is seen by a physiotherapist on the day of surgery, it is proposed that they will be discharged from hospital sooner. This benefits the patient (they return to daily function quicker) and staff (lessens demand for hospital beds).

Aim: To increase the possibility of a physiotherapist being able to see a post-operative total hip or knee replacement patient on the day of surgery (day 0), in line with the ERP.

Actions – What changes can you make that will result in the improvement you seek

What are the steps you plan to take or have taken to address the need for improvement including stakeholder/colleague involvement and specific activities/actions?

- Surgical operations for all patients on the ERP to take place before midday.
- Every Monday (the busiest day of the week for operations), one physiotherapist will work between 17:00 and 20:00.
- A decision will be made regarding the feasibility of the changes.
- If agreed, a physiotherapist rota will be organised for the Monday evening shift.
- A pilot trail will take place for one month and its effectiveness will be reviewed.
- If successful (and practical), the ERP modifications will be introduced permanently.

Impact – Measurement – How will you know that a change is an improvement?

What is the change your improvement activities should make or have made for patients, carers, staff or the service, including any specific indicators or measures of that change?

- Length of post-operative hospital duration, comparing ERP to non-ERP.
- Feedback from physiotherapists involved in the ERP.
- Patient feedback and satisfaction with treatment.

REFLECTIONS

What went well?

- The orthopaedic physiotherapy team all agreed that the ERP had its faults.
- The team were pleased that I came up with a solution to address the main ERP shortfall.
- Greatly received by the majority of patients, that is if they were seen earlier.

Who did you involve? (patient/service-user/colleagues/multidisciplinary team [MDT])

- Discussion with my educator and orthopaedic physiotherapy colleagues.
- Liaised with the lead ERP physiotherapist.
- Received feedback from post-operative patients on the ERP.

Did the improvement link to any current improvement programmes in your placement setting?

- The ERP has been recently introduced to aim to decrease a patient's duration in hospital following a joint replacement.
- This service improvement proposal aimed to slightly modify the current programme, to improve its efficiency/successfulness.

Were there any issues/constraints?

- Is it possible for surgeons to routinely operate on patients on the ERP in the morning?
- It may not always be the time of surgery that influences the time the patient arrives back on the ward. Duration in the recovery area also has an impact.
- Staffing levels and costs in respect of working an evening shift on Monday.
- Not ALL joint replacement operations take place on Monday. What would happen on the other weekdays?

Did the team agree to take your ideas forward?

Not during my placement time in the orthopaedic team. Although, the team were keen to put forward the idea in the future.

Case study 2

Name: Speech & Language Therapy Student
Placement Type: Children's Nurseries

Background – This should include your aim (what you are trying to accomplish)

Give a description of the problem and your identification of the need for improvement including any implications for patients, carers and staff.

There are two different nurseries within this region that have been targeted to use MAKATON (a language programme using signs, symbols and speech to help people communicate) in the past. This has not been successful in generalisation, especially with the training used and resources given. Signs and symbols have been pasted around the nurseries but not many staff use them, leaving them redundant. If staff were using the signs and symbols, it was to greatly varying degrees.

If MAKATON was implemented within the nursery, it would improve the communication between both children and staff, especially considering that there are children in both nurseries which use this as a main means of communication. There are also high rates of bilingualism within the nurseries, which indicates the need for a common means of communication. There will be fewer barriers between children who have different needs, also improving their social integration. Parents may also find this effective and it has been shown to improve speech and language development amongst children. Children generally use both the MAKATON signs and speech – parents do not need to worry that using MAKATON could affect their child's speech.

Actions – What changes can you make that will result in the improvement you seek?

What are the steps you plan to take or have taken to address the need for improvement including stakeholder/colleague involvement and specific activities/actions?

- Communicate with nurseries to encourage them to take part in new MAKATON training to help implementation in the environment.
- Teach and model how Pictoys packs can be used alongside MAKATON in both the nurseries and at home (to help generalisation).
- More games and songs that use MAKATON will be demonstrated.
- Encourage staff to cascade the information to their colleagues if they cannot attend the training.
- Give resources, including two copies of each sign, to the nurseries to avoid them being forgotten.
- Request feedback on the training so that further improvement can be made in the future.

Impact – Measurement – How will you know that a change is an improvement?

What is the change your improvement activities should make or have made for patients, carers, staff or the service, including any specific indicators or measures of that change?

The nurseries will be receiving more resources than previously that encourage the use of MAKATON and are easily accessible. Duplicate signs will also be provided so that fewer are lost or forgotten (these were also laminated so that they were not ruined).

Speech and Language Therapists need the nursery to use MAKATON and have requested that we do the training. Therefore, they will be able to observe and record the outcomes and judge if they are effective.

Due to MAKATON now being implemented, there is a common means of communication used that children enjoy. This further encourages the use of it and members of staff always have resources available. Any new members of staff will be able to access training materials that will be given to the nursery.

REFLECTIONS

What went well?

The majority of staff were enthusiastic at the training and were willing to learn. Staff members were keen to be left with resources after the first training session so that they could start trying to use it.

Who did you involve? (patient/user/colleague/MDT)

Nursery staff (including the Special Educational Needs Coordinator) and children who attended the nurseries. Speech and Language Therapists were also involved in the planning of the training and will be included within following up the nurseries afterwards.

Did the improvement link to any current improvement programmes in your placement setting?

The improvement was suggested to us by Speech and Language Therapists that currently work with the nurseries after a previous training session did not produce the results they wanted. Using the cascade training meant that it was more cost effective for the nurseries.

Were there any issues/constraints?

- Not all staff could attend training sessions.
- Some training environments were difficult and distracting.
- Not all members of staff wanted to take part.
- We could only provide three sessions, of which the nurseries could only have two due to half-term.
- Due to the nurseries being short staffed, it was very difficult to find the time and environment to carry out the training.

Did the team agree to take your ideas forward?

- Management of both nurseries were very keen for their staff to implement MAKATON.
- Due to their motivation and interest, they were more encouraged to use it with the children in different settings.
- With new resources, staff thought it would be easier to generalise.
- The staff requested extra symbols that they thought would be useful.

Case study 3
Name: Occupational Therapy Student
Placement Type: Spinal Injuries Unit

Background – This should include your aim (what you are trying to accomplish)

Give a description of the problem and your identification of the need for improvement including any implications for patients, carers and staff.

There were no social activities incorporated into the in-patient timetable. After discussion with the MDT, I found that they were aiming to organise an activity for all the patients to engage in.

There appeared to be no element of socialising for the patients and my aim is to encourage this aspect through the various activities offered.

I aim to plan weekly activities, for example the Wii, pool, outings, educational programmes and so on with the help of the Occupational Therapy assistant.

The level of supervision required will depend on the number of patients and their level of spinal cord lesion.

Budgeting will also determine the type of activity permitted.

Actions – What changes can you make that will result in the improvement you seek?

What are the steps you plan to take or have taken to address the need for improvement including stakeholder/colleague involvement and specific activities/actions?

- I held discussions with the MDT to find out what they hoped to achieve by carrying out organised activities for patients.
- I spoke to the patients to find out what their interests were and whether we could incorporate them into future sessions under a budget.
- I set out weekly activity sessions and booked these into late afternoon slots and this was agreed with by all MDT. This was to ensure that:
  - Patients would have a suitable length of time for maximum participation in the activity.
  - The activity would not compromise any other therapy sessions.
  - All activities will be working within a budget and using the resources in the hospital.

Impact – Measurement – How will you know that a change is an improvement?

What is the change your improvement activities should make or have made for patients, carers, staff or the service, including any specific indicators or measures of that change?

- I will supply a comment sheet after each activity so patients have a means by which to express their opinions as to what went well, not so well, improvements and so on. Also, they will be actively encouraged to verbalise these comments, especially if they are unable to write.

This is a qualitative approach.

- As a measurement tool I could carry out the Likert Scale to monitor what the patients thought of the activity. These results are quantifiable.

REFLECTIONS

What went well?

- I felt all aspects went well; the preparatory phases were difficult at times as problem solving was important for maximum participation by the patients and to keep coming up with new ideas.
- I enjoyed speaking to the patients about their preferences and their reactions of enjoyment were priceless and I felt I added to their rehabilitation.
- One comment was that they felt using a wheelchair in the community was vital in returning to a normal way of life.

Who did you involve? (patient/user/colleague/MDT)

We actively encouraged all patients to participate but this was not mandatory. Any colleague could help supervise or join in; this was easier when the activities were based on the hospital grounds.

Did the improvement link to any current improvement programmes in your placement setting?

No.

Were there any issues/constraints?

- The budget was a constraint, at times the activity sessions involved going on outings.
- I had to be creative with my ideas and ask the patients/MDT for any ideas so as to build up a portfolio of activity sessions.
- No other issues were raised.

Did the team agree to take your ideas forward?

Yes, the team have agreed to take my ideas forward. It was also very helpful that the MDT had been given approval to carry out therapeutic activities with patients as part of their therapy timetable.

Potential interview questions in this area

Experience:

- What personal experience do you have of service improvement in the workplace?
- Supplementary: Can you provide any real examples of where you have contributed to service improvement?

Knowledge:
- How would you decide where there is a need for service improvement?
- Supplementary: How would go about implementing improvements within this job role?

Skills/Behaviours:
- How might you go about implementing service improvement and what skills does this demonstrate?
- Supplementary: Can you provide examples of how you have demonstrated these skills?

Insight/Influence/Leadership:
- What do you think causes people to be resistant to change and why is this the case?
- Supplementary: How would you go about encouraging people to make improvements?

References

Adair J (2012) *Effective Innovation.* London: Pan.

Darzi Lord A (2008) *High quality care for all.* London: Crown Publications.

DoH (Department of Health) (2004) *The Knowledge and Skills Framework (NHS KSF) and the Development Review Process.* London: Department of Health Publications.

DoH (Department of Health) (2013a) *The NHS Constitution.* London: Crown Publications: London.

DoH (Department of Health) (2013b) *Making the NHS more efficient and less bureaucratic.* (https://www.gov.uk/government/publications/2010-to-2015-government-policy-nhs-efficiency/2010-to-2015-government-policy-nhs-efficiency; last accessed 18 August 2015).

Francis R (2013) *Report of the Mid Staffordshire NHS Foundation Trust Public Inquiry,* Executive summary. Available at https://www.gov.uk/government/uploads/system/uploads/attachment_data/file/279124/0947.pdf; last accessed 18 August 2015.

Harvey L, Plimmer L, Moon S and Geall V (1997) *Student satisfaction manual.* Buckingham, UK: Open University Press.

Hillage J and Pollard E (1998) *Employability: developing a framework for policy analysis.* Research Report RR85. London: Department for Education and Employment.

Hunt B (2010) *The history and simplicity of lean process improvement.* Available at http://www.processexcellencenetwork.com/lean-six-sigma-business-transformation/articles/the-history-and-simplicity-of-lean-process-improve/; last accessed 10 August 2015.

Langley GJ, Moen R, Nolan KM *et al.* (1996) *The improvement guide: A practical approach to enhancing organizational performance.* San Francisco, CA: Jossey-Bass.

Lansley A (2010) *QIPP: Quality, Innovation,* Productivity and Prevention, Available at http://webarchive.nationalarchives.gov.uk/+/www.dh.gov.uk/en/Aboutus/Chiefprofessionalofficers/Chiefnursingofficer/Energiseforexcellence/DH_121229; last accessed 10 August 2015.

Larner J (2012a) *The yellow brick road to improvement.* Poster presented at the International Forum for Safety and Quality in Healthcare 2012, Paris.
Larner J (2012b) *The service improvement task: How I feel it enhances my employability.* Poster presented at the UEA School of Allied Health Professions Employment Symposium, 9 2012b, Norwich, UK.
Larner J and Collier J (2012) *Chapter 12: Tools for service improvement.* In CS Hong and D Harrison, *Tools for continuing professional development.* London: Quay Books.
Lees D (2002) *Graduate Employability – Literature Review.* Available at http://www.qualityresearchinternational.com/esecttools/esectpubs/leeslitreview.pdf; last accessed 10 August 2015.
Lister S, Larner J and Lynch M (2011) *Ten thousand students undertake improvement projects: The experience of increasing improvement capability in the healthcare workforce by supporting the introduction of service improvement into pre-qualification curriculum of healthcare professionals.* Poster presented at the International Forum for Quality and Safety in Healthcare 2013, Amsterdam.
Little B (2001) Reading between the lines of graduate employability. *Quality in Higher Education,* 7(2):121–129.
Lowden K, Hall S, Elliot D and Lewin J (2011) *Employers' perceptions of the employability skills of new graduates.* University of Glasgow, commissioned and published by the Edge Foundation.
NHS Employers (2010) *Summary descriptions of core KSF dimensions.* Available at http://www.nhsemployers.org/~/media/Employers/Documents/SiteCollectionDocuments/Summary_KSF_core_dim_fb131110.docx; last accessed 18 August 2015.
NHS Leadership Academy (2011) *The NHS Leadership Framework, NHS Institution for Innovation and Improvement: Warwick,* UK: Warwick University.
NHSI (National Health Service Institute for Innovation and Improvement) (2007) *Process mapping, analysis and redesign, General improvement skills, Improvement Leaders Guide.* Nottingham, UK: NHSI Publications.
NHSI (National Health Service Institute for Innovation and Improvement) (2008) *Improvement in pre-registration education for better, safer healthcare.* Nottingham, UK: NHSI Publications.
Scally G and Donaldson L (1998) Clinical governance and the drive for quality improvement in the new NHS in England. *BMJ;* **317**:61. (Available at: 10.1136/bmj.317.7150.61; last accessed 10 August 2015.)
Skills for Health (2014) *The employability skills matrix for health.* Available at http://www.skillsforhealth.org.uk/resources/search?searchword=Employability+skills+matrix+for+health; last accessed 19 August 2015.
Worth R (2011) *Beat the cuts.* St. Albans, UK: Ecademy Press.

Chapter 7 **Business skills**

David Dowdeswell-Allaway
Norwich, UK

If you want to build a career in the health sector, regardless of your feelings about business, you will need to engage with business jargon, processes and approaches in order to survive and, hopefully, thrive. That does not mean that you have to compromise your values – there are those that feel that health and business values are incommensurable – rather, engaging with business approaches can strengthen the provision of health services at all levels, from sole trader to business unit within a large hospital. In addition, there is a growing sector of businesses known as 'social enterprises' that differ from traditional profit-centred businesses. These jargon terms will be defined as we progress through this chapter.

One aspect necessary in understanding business is getting to know the jargon. 'Sole trader', 'business unit' and 'social enterprise' are examples of jargon that we shall translate into straight forward terms in this chapter. As well as demystifying 'business speak', this chapter will break business into four broad areas:

1. Things
2. People
3. Time
4. Money.

Each area will be developed to address the following:

1. **Things.** Under this vague heading are the:
   a. *Legal structures* that define a business, the choices available and the rationale behind each of the choices.
   b. *Marketing* of things, whether services or products.
   c. *Assets*, the physical things that your business owns.
2. **People.** This section will outline the wide range of people, or *stakeholders*, that any business needs to attend to:
   a. In-facing: recruitment, training, management.
   b. Out-facing: customers, funders, regulatory authorities.

How to Develop Your Healthcare Career: A Guide to Employability and Professional Development, First Edition. Edited by Lisa Taylor.
© 2016 John Wiley & Sons, Ltd. Published 2016 by John Wiley & Sons, Ltd.

    c. Management structures and frameworks.

    d. Communication, appraisal, goals, discipline, motivation.

3. **Time.** This section deals with the only non-variable that you will need to master using:

    1. Goals

    2. Planning

    3. Strategy

4. **Money.** This must be made, one way or another, even if you are working in a not-for-profit business. Keeping track of your money – goods and/or services bought and sold – as well as understanding how to raise money for strategic developments, is vital. Hence:

    1. Income and expenditure

    2. Accounting

    3. Tax and VAT

    4. Sales.

Of course, all four of these interlink in myriad cause–effect relationships but looking, briefly, at each in turn may help to demystify the term 'business' and give you the means by which you can begin to think about your life experiences, to date, through a business lens. This, in turn, will help you to articulate your experiences in the discourse of business for the purpose of entering into business yourself, whether that be through the job application process, or moving into a junior business position, or setting yourself up in a business of your own, or with one, or two, trusted others. In other words, *how to build a career in the health sector.*

Things

Any business needs a legal base, it needs to sell something and it needs to buy things. Consequently, this vague term is been broken down here into three areas: legal, marketing and assets. How can knowledge of these things help you to build your career? Let us look at these three areas and then ask that question more specifically at various points throughout this chapter.

Legal structures

The thing that makes a business a 'business' is its legal structure. Without such legal structure business-as-a-verb carries on (e.g. black market trading and bartering) but business-as-an-entity cannot. It is within business-as-an-entity that the business activity can legitimately be carried out. There are a specific set of business legal structures that you will have encountered and, therefore, use both as models for your reflection on 'business' and models upon which you can build your career. There are two main names for businesses. In the United

States of America the main term for a business is 'corporation' (from the Latin, *corpus*, meaning 'body'). In the United Kingdom the synonym is 'company' (from Old French, *compagnie*, meaning group of people). For the basis of this chapter, I shall use the term 'company'.

There are, in the United Kingdom, four basic types of business (the United States equivalents are based on the same distinctions).

1. Sole trader
2. Limited company
3. Partnership
4. Social enterprise.

Sole trader

- As a sole trader, you run your own business as an individual. You can keep all your business's profits after you have paid tax on them.
- You can employ staff. 'Sole trader' means you're responsible for the business, not that you have to work alone.
- You are personally responsible for any losses your business makes.' (https://www.gov.uk/business-legal-structures/sole-trader)

Health workers, such as peripatetic physiotherapists or private nurses, are often sole traders. The main advantage of being a sole trader (self-employed) is that what you earn belongs to you. The flip side, of course, is that what you lose belongs to you too. As a sole trader you will need to file your own tax returns to your country's government and, in the United Kingdom, pay your National Insurance (which is a form of tax that is specifically linked to the UK Social Security system; https://www.gov.uk/national-insurance/overview).

Limited company

- A limited company is an organisation that you can set up to run your business [through].
- It is responsible in its own right [as if it were a person] for everything it does and its finances are separate to your personal finances.
- Any profit it makes is owned by the company, after it pays Corporation Tax [to the UK Government]. The company can then share its profits. (https://www.gov.uk/business-legal-structures/limited-company)

The advantage of a limited company over being a sole trader is that should the business fail your personal wealth and possessions (e.g. your house) are protected. As a sole trader your home may be sold to pay off your company's debts. There are more bureaucratic demands involved in running a Limited Company but in the UK the online help at www.gov.uk is very good. The 'limited' refers to the ownership of the company being limited to its shareholders. A shareholder is a person that has bought a share of the company. A simple limited company, in the United Kingdom, can have one owner that owns all the shares, or it can have many owners, each of whom owns a number of shares. Very large organisations may sell their shares to the public via, for example, the London Stock Exchange or the USA NASDAQ (http://www.companieshouse.gov.uk). If you set up a business you will be known as the Company Director. You will need to file your own tax returns as well as your Corporation Tax returns (your personal tax and your company's tax) and use a Pay As You Earn (PAYE) system if you pay yourself a salary. In large companies, profit is divided up and paid out to its shareholders as a 'dividend'. As a Director, you can receive dividends in addition to your salary.

Partnership

A common form of company within the health sector in the United Kingdom is that of the General Practice, many of which are called a 'partnership'. There are two main types of partnership. In an 'Ordinary' Partnership, in which the partners each take responsibility for the success and failure of the business, profits are shared between the partners, and each partner files their own tax return. A Limited Partnership shares the liability for debts among the partners. A Limited Liability Partnership is a business in which each partner's liability for debt is limited to the amount that they have invested in the company. There are some bureaucratic distinctions between a Limited Company and a Partnership. (For more information see, e.g., https://www.gov.uk/business-legal-structures/limited-partnership-and-limited-liability-partnership.)

Social enterprise

A 'social enterprise' is a business that 'helps people or communities [and has] social, charitable or community-based objectives' (https://www.gov.uk/set-up-a-social-enterprise). There are some specific legal structures for the social enterprise sector, though sole traders, limited companies and limited partnerships can be social enterprises. Specialist legal structures in the United Kingdom are charitable incorporated organisation(CIO), co-operative, industrial and provident society (https://www.gov.uk/set-up-a-social-enterprise). It is the business objectives that set a social enterprise apart from other businesses. They came to prominence within the health sector as part of the UK Conservative/Liberal Democrat coalition government's theme of the 'big society' (Cabinet Office, 2010) and within the NHS this was aimed at the dramatic increase within the NHS of staff-owned (mutual) companies. The debate over this decision is beyond the scope of this brief introduction though.

What may be useful for you, at this point of your career, is to understand that the common themes underlying most forms of social enterprise are that they:

- Have a clear social and/or environmental mission set out in their governing documents.
- Generate the majority of their income through trade.
- Reinvest the majority of their profits.

- Be autonomous of state.
- Be majority controlled in the interests of the social mission.
- Be accountable and transparent.
  (http://www.socialenterprise.org.uk/about/about-social-enterprise)
  A useful, but by no means exclusive, definition of social enterprise is:

> *'Business ventures that prioritize [sic] their social purpose(s), operate ethically and promote democratic ownership and governance by primary stakeholders.'*

(http://www.socialenterpriseeurope.co.uk/what-is-social-enterprise/)

Time for reflection

How can knowledge of these things help you to build your career? Take a moment to think of the last business that you engaged with (e.g. where you work, a local shop, an online provider of a good or service) and identify what type of legal structure it likely has. Why might it have that structure? What benefits may that structure have for that specific business?

Marketing

Marketing is essential if your business is going to attract customers. Marketing exists in obvious ways, such as advertising your product or service on a web site. It is also fundamental for health promotion. Note that marketing also takes place at an individual level; you market yourself at a job interview. So what are the themes common among these disparate examples that are worth you paying attention to as you build your career?

Marketing is:

- a management process;
- it is about the exchange of goods and services;
- it anticipates and meets consumer's needs;
- it creates profits.
  (http://media3.bournemouth.ac.uk/marketing/02defining/02defining.html)

It is easy to see how this set of distinctions applies to the marketing of your businesses products or services. You have to manage how that happens, your efforts lead to the exchange of your products or services for, normally, money, your marketing looks into the future and responds to your customers' needs, and your efforts generate income sufficient not only to pay your salary but also to satisfy other stakeholders that support you in exchange for payment, such as shareholders or members.

When you apply marketing principles to applying for a new job, again you need to manage the process (you cannot just leave it to chance), you need to display your skills, attitudes, experience and values (your offer) in exchange for the job, which means that you have to anticipate what the organisation to which you are applying needs and convince them that you will contribute to making a profit for the business. This holds true whether you are applying to work for a profit-driven business or a social enterprise.

Time for reflection

How can knowledge of these things help you to build your career?

1. Think of an advertisement that sticks in your mind. What were the key strengths of the product or service being advertised? What values are communicated about the business marketing the product or service?

2. Think about you marketing yourself to a potential employer or business partner. What values are communicated about you through your self-marketing?

Sales and customer relationships

If marketing is what is required to get a product or service known to potential customers, all businesses must then sell these things to customers and also build a relationship with its customers, so that they come back again and again.

The notion of 'selling' can be distasteful for some people; however, we have all sold things all our lives. What is an infant up to when it cries and cries? It is selling the parent or caregiver the idea that some food would be good, now! When you understand that we need the same skills to sell an idea or a car you may begin to appreciate your existing selling skills. Whether your business is selling antibacterial cleaning agents, or selling the idea of healthy eating, the skills are the same. You will need to develop a clear and appealing image of the product, service or idea, outline the benefits to committing to it, and 'close the deal'. In other words, get a person to say 'Yes' and to hand over the cash, sign the contract or set out new life changes.

Time for reflection

How can knowledge of these things help you to build your career?

• What was the last physical product that you bought? What sales and customer relationship activities can you identify from that experience?

• Remember, now, the last time that you were a service user of a health service. How does that experience compare to that from your shopping experience?

• When you next apply for a job think of it as a process of 'selling yourself' to a 'customer' that is your potential employer. Using the ideas from the paragraph, above, what kind of image can you create for yourself? What will you bring to the customer that will make you an appealing prospect? How can you get the customer to say 'Yes, I will employ you?'. Notice how you feel, having read those questions. For some people entering the health services, such questions raise uncomfortable, even antagonistic feelings, since they can give rise to self-talk such as 'But I'm not a product, I'm a human being that wants to care for people, not money'. Fair enough, and the two are not incompatible. Adopting the mind-set of business can be useful at times for all of us. All parents will have excellent sales techniques developed through persuading a young child to eat. What do you need to develop to sell better?

Assets

Assets are things that belong to your business. Assets are either tangible or intangible. *Tangible assets* are things such as the machines, buildings and equipment necessary for your business to run. Tangible assets are not consumed in the delivery of your service. For example, an ultrasound machine is an asset but the water-based lubricant is not. Tangible assets appear on your balance sheet [see the section on Accounts] and can be sold to raise money if necessary.

Intangible assets are not physical things and they do not appear on your balance sheet. Instead, they are things like your, or your businesses', reputation, market presence or intellectual property. Intellectual property is the term for all things such as logos, brands, patents and trademarks that help identify your business or define your products or services (https://www.gov.uk/intellectual-property-an-overview/overview).

People

1. Stakeholders
   a. In-facing: recruitment, training and management including appraisal, goals, discipline.
   b. Out-facing: customers, funders, regulatory authorities.
2. Management structures and frameworks.
3. Communication.

Stakeholders

Regardless of whether you work in the public or private sector, within an independent business unit, a business unit within a large institutional structure or alone, you are going to have to work with people. All of the people that you have to work with, or for, are called your 'stakeholders'. As such, they all have some claim on your time and attention. One of the skills that you can develop throughout your career is identifying which group of stakeholders get your attention at which times.

It can be very helpful to spend a while identifying the stakeholders in various contexts in order for you to develop the ability to articulate, in a straightforward way, the complex arrangement of people that a business unit has to deal with. Imagine an interview question, perhaps whilst in the final year of your degree, 'Think of the dental practice (supermarket, café, cinema etc.) that you use; who are the stakeholders?' Your ability to answer this type of question in an orderly and inclusive way demonstrates your breadth of awareness of the people involved.

So who are these stakeholders? It can be easiest to begin by dividing stakeholders into two broad groups, sometimes known as 'in-facing' or 'inward facing' and 'out-facing' or 'outward facing'. These terms refer to those stakeholders that pay attention to the inside of the business, in-facing: directors/partners, employees, contractors and so on, and those whose attention is on the outside of the business, out-facing: customers, patients, shareholders and so on. Regardless of the size of your business unit, these two broad categories remain the same; the difference comes only in terms of scale and category. It is worth remembering that your own family can be considered as stakeholders, since how your business goes – time that you spend at work, work load, income and so on – will affect how you relate to members of your family.

In-facing

There are, of course, many ways to slice the stakeholder pie after we have stuffed it with the complete set of stakeholders. Remember, what is important to you, with your business hat on, is who should you be paying attention to right now? Have you had the experience of receiving excellent customer service? Where was the other person's attention then? On you. Poor customer service typically means that their attention is anywhere but you. Things that you will need to pay attention to, at varying points of your career, will be the in-facing functions of recruitment, training and management (discussed in the later '*Communication*' section).

Out-facing

As you enter business, it is worth paying attention to your customers, whether they are an obvious customer, for example a person handing over cash for a product or service, or a less obvious customer, for example another business unit within the large organisation that you work for. Regardless of who your customer is, it is reasonable to accept that each customer demands the same high-quality service that you would expect from someone providing you with a product or service. Again, think back to your own experiences of being paid attention to as you received excellent customer service. As you deal with your patient, your accountant, your supplier, your administrators, you will get the best from them if you pay them quality attention. In your role you will, at times, need to be in-facing and pay attention to the people that help your business to succeed. At other times, out-facing and pay attention to those people that give you the money to help your business to succeed.

Just because you have chosen to work in the health sector, as opposed, say, to the retail sector, does not mean that you can pay less attention to your whole range of stakeholders - internal and external - than can the in-store salesperson.

Time for reflection

How can knowledge of these things help you to build your career? Think back on your academic career. As you do, identify the stakeholders from the view of:
1. The university
2. A lecturer
3. A student.

Management structures and skills

Even if you do, or intend to, work alone, you will still benefit from understanding management skills because you need to manage your things: yourself, your time and your money. However, it is more common to associate management structures, in conjunction with management skills, in the business setting involving some, or many, people.

Many jobs in the health sector involve some aspect of supervision or management, so some knowledge of these things can benefit you greatly, even if your main focus of attention will be on your patients. Refer back to the section on stakeholders and remember that you will need to pay attention to people in a variety of settings, not just those that are the obvious benefactors of your attention, such as your patients.

Management structures need to be designed to manage the *things, people, time* and *money*. Already, you may see that any management structure will have at least these four segments. There are myriad models of management structure (a quick search on www.amazon.co.uk returned nearly 60 000 items under the search term 'management structure'). What this means for you is that you will benefit from some study of management structures that are one or two steps ahead of your current level of complexity. I recommend that for now, you apply the simple, four segment approach to the divination of management structures that you currently interact with.

Time for reflection
How can knowledge of these things help you to build your career?
Identify a business and its structure according to the four segments of *things, people, time, money* that have been used here.

Business planning

To help you develop the necessary skills involved in understanding management structures, it can be useful to begin by using business planning software. Such software is commonly freely available from high street banks and will help you to identify those aspects of a business that you know, or are interesting in creating, in a detailed, structured way. Every business or business unit ought to have a business plan because this will help you identify your stakeholders, your in-facing and out-facing foci of attention, and necessary information for the setting up and maintenance and development of your business.

Something that is a common problem for small and medium-sized businesses is long-term planning; their focus is normally on the present or short term. A business plan forces you take a longer view and plan to reach certain goals that you deem appropriate to your personal, or business, development.

Marketing (again)

I have already mentioned that marketing is an essential part of any business, regardless of size, but it is worth reiterating here that for any business to succeed it needs to have the ability to completely and utterly focus upon the needs and wants of its customers. This applies both to external and internal customers.

HR management

Working alone does not exist. If you are engaged in business then you have stakeholders to whom you must pay attention at different times. Your in-facing focus will need, at some time, to include the management duties of people management and, possibly, formal human resource (HR) management. The basic functions of people management include the setting of goals for each person, or group of people, to strive for, the motivation of people to engage with their work and, hopefully, to enjoy it, and the monitoring of people to comply with necessary standards, laws and regulations.

Communication

Here are a few aspects of communication that can prove useful to you as you build your career:

- You cannot not-communicate. Even silence says something to those witnessing it. If you remember this as you also pay attention to which of your stakeholders needs your attention in the here-and-now, then you will already be building your reputation as a quality provider of your service.

• Feedback is just information. It is information about the person giving the feedback (what they have been paying attention to) as much as it is about you.

The most useful model that I have encountered is called the Johari Window (Figure 7.1) (Luft and Ingham, 1955).

You can apply the Johari model to an individual or a business. The basic idea is that you seek to extend the public area as an individual because in developing your career you need to seek information about your performance (feedback) and you need to let your coworkers, managers, clients know something about you (disclosure) in order to build trust, identify training needs and set goals. As a business, much the same applies. We often hear about the need for 'transparency' in our health services and, using the Johari Window as a model, that means reducing the hidden through disclosure. In the United Kingdom, disclosure can be forced through law but the truth is better received, and more quickly forgiven, if it is offered. Businesses must seek information about their finances, their market position, their customers

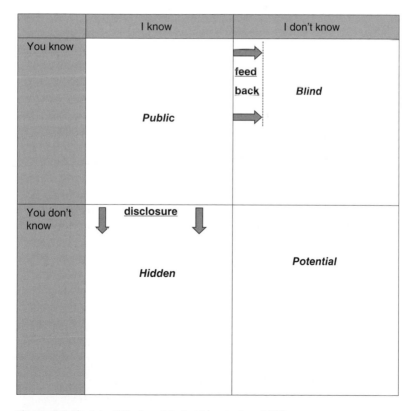

Figure 7.1 The Johari Window. Adapted from Ingham 1955

and so on and they will dedicate time and money to gather such feedback in order to shrink the blind section of the Johari Window. For both the individual and the business, the Johari Window suggests that through disclosure and feedback potential is released.

Here are a few uses for paying attention to how you communicate as an individual and a business (remember, as you build your career, your developing insight into communication in both individual and business contexts will be valuable):

- Marketing
- Professional development
- Human resource development
- Recruitment
- Training
- Management.

Communication for marketing

Marketing demands the collection of information (communication into the business) before creating messages to increase awareness of your products and services (communication out from the business). As an individual, you will need to be skilled at selling your ideas to management, as, in the face of tight budget controls, each idea needs to be sold on its merits, so being able to construct a clear message is more likely to lead to your idea being accepted.

Communication for professional development

Businesses and individuals develop and strengthen through communication with other people and businesses (see the Johari Window, Figure 7.1). As a health professional you will likely be compelled to engage with continuing professional development (CPD) of some sort, but this should not be considered solely in the realm of technical knowledge. The exchange of ideas, the sharing of experience, the human interaction of groups, networks, fora, and conferences are all available means of communication that can add to your development and to that of your business. In building your career, your ability to demonstrate your engagement with others to support your learning will be highly valued in interview settings.

Communication for human resource development (HRD)

One of the dangers of jargonising human experience is that it can dehumanise how one person relates to another. In the health professions a person seeking help is called a 'patient': that is helpful jargon in many contexts, but in some contexts remembering that that patient has a name, and using their name, can make a huge difference. Calling the people that you work with a 'human resource', in my experience, has no value other than for making difficult decisions easier, as it is emotionally easier to 'reduce the budget for HR' than to face 'having to make people redundant'. Lasting businesses, especially those whose chief stakeholders are individuals, as in the health sector, rely on building relationships between people. If you can remember this as you move into higher management positions then you are more likely to maintain a level of humanity to support your decisions and how you communicate them to the individuals that are your stakeholders.

Communication for recruitment

What was the toughest interview question that you have had? Now consider that you may be responsible for taking on staff: Would you ask that same question? What is the employer searching for through each question asked? What do you want to know before investing in a new employee? Did you realise that when you take on a new employee you are not only going to have to pay them at least the minimum wage, but also certain taxes (e.g. National Insurance in the UK), training costs, employers liability insurance, consider sickness payments, maternity/paternity leave, changes to the work infrastructure (where are they going to sit?), what about their pension?, and have you thought of the cost of your time in managing them? Before you start looking for a new employee, you need to be able to answer all of these questions. Once you have done that, be clear about the duties that you want the person to fulfil and how you will measure their speed of progress to becoming as autonomous as you would like them to be.

Communication for training

The Johari Window shows where your communication will be really necessary: in the feedback area. You cannot expect a person to change their behaviour unless they are given behaviour-specific feedback. Employees and colleagues are not mind readers. If you appreciate what a person does, tell them. If you do not like what a person does, tell them. Remember the key point about feedback: *it is just information*. That means that you describe the behaviour and you do not judge the person. Your noticing of what your employees are doing that is not up to your expected standard is called, in HR jargon, a 'training needs analysis'. There are many models for this (good examples can be found at: http://www.cipd.co.uk/toolclicks/learning/training-tools/training-needs-analysis/identify-data-needs-collection/default.aspx). Once complete, training can be arranged or procured, goals set and a timetable for achievement laid out. This takes us to the last of the needs for communication set out here.

Communication for management

Whether you manage only one person, or many, your ability to communicate clearly will be vital. Be clear about whether you are communicating because things are going as you would like them to be, or if they are not. If things are going well, how can you communicate that such that good practice continues or even spreads? How can you make staff feel valued when they do well? Remember when you have felt appreciated: How did you know that you were? If things are not going as you would like them to, remember to identify the specific behaviour that needs to change, and to communicate clear behaviour-based feedback that a person can follow. Only by providing that feedback will you be in a position to monitor progress and, if it is not forthcoming, begin disciplinary processes. As an employer, there are many legal protections for employees and if you do not communicate clearly, set reviews for progress and clear targets then you will be on thin ice if you attempt to discipline an employee. Good management communication needs to be simply stated (please avoid management jargon, examples of which can be found at http://www.buzzwords4u.co.uk/).

Jargon is only of use to those that understand it and they are always in-facing. A 'stool' for a doctor is normally very different from a 'stool' for your kitchen! As you develop your communication skills through your career it can be most helpful for you to speak the truth simply and in terms that your listener(s) can understand; you will be respected for it. Never assume that the people that your business serves will understand the jargon of your business. Train all out-facing staff to talk in jargon-free language.

Time for reflection

How can knowledge of these things help you to build your career? Visit the web site http://www.buzzwords4u.co.uk/ and translate a few of the phrases into simple, straightforward language. As you rehearse your answers to the suggested interview questions at the end of this chapter, check for straightforwardness in your answers. Also, check the questions for possible jargon.

Time

You cannot make time, only use it wisely. You will have approximately 1700 hours of work in one year. How you divide your time between your duties, your in-facing and out-facing stakeholders, and your own mental and physical health is of prime importance. If you review how you divided your time as a child, then as a student, you will recognise patterns that are very likely to be with you throughout your career. This may be good news. However, if you recognise deficiencies in your management of time and your organisation, perhaps you can dedicate some time to learning how to do things differently.

Time management and organisation

Time management and being organised are essential business skills. You already have much of what is needed or else you would not be reading these words. All time management is, is the deliberate assignation of packets of time to specific duties. There are many and varied models designed to help you with this: grids, matrixes, tables and charts (Blanchard and Johnson, 2004; Covey, 1989; Zeller, 2008) though most of them will do much the same thing, namely: firstly, identify your stakeholders: secondly, identify your duties; thirdly, rate each according to priority and importance.

Time for reflection

How can knowledge of these things help you to build your career?

1. Use tomorrow as your context.
2. Identify all the stakeholders involved in tomorrow.
3. Identify all of your duties tomorrow (eat, sleep, excrete, work, play).
4. Rank each item identified in point 3, with one being the most important.
5. Assign one of three colours to each of the stakeholders identified in point 2 – Green = good relationship, Orange = relationship needs some attention, Red = relationship needs urgent attention.
6. Draw out this chart, with you in the centre, the most important stakeholder closest to you, the least important furthest from you. Finally, draw a line between you and each stakeholder of the appropriate colour from step 5.
7. Review your chart: imagine that you are in a management position. What actions would you take? What would you prioritise? What would you advise another person to do facing tomorrow's chart? What does this say about you? (e.g. would you instruct a subordinate to take the same actions as you would take yourself?) Where do your priorities lie? Do you need to take urgent action? What two-week, two-month, two-year plans can you make?

Setting goals

Goal setting is one area of time management that we shall focus on here. Without having specifics to focus on, to aim for, to set in the future, we are, literally, aimless. Any business that has no goals will fail. Imagine a shop that had no goals for re-stocking its shelves; it would wait until the shelves were empty before ordering more stock and its customers would go elsewhere. 'Vision' is the term often used in managerial settings for the ultimate goal of a business. As you build your career it can be useful to break your goals into achievable steps and to set regular times to review your progress towards your ultimate success, or re-writing of your goals. Setting goals for your staff is vital. As a follow-up to the Johari Window, goal setting can be an excellent way to target the achievement of goals related to specific feedback. Remember, if you do not give others specific information on what you do not like, you cannot expect them to change.

The most common form of goal setting is known as SMART, with the acronym representing the need for goals to be: Specific enough to be able to Measure, Achievable and Realistic and, finally, Time-bound (there are many variations on this acronym; Rubin, 2002). In my experience of setting goals with individuals and organisations, I have found adding some questions enhances the likelihood of people pursuing their goals and, therefore, I encourage you to ask yourself questions such as:

- What do you want to have happen? (If you answer with a negative, e.g., 'I want to stop worrying', turn it into a positive goal by asking yourself, 'What do I want instead of worrying?').
- What is currently in your control?
- When, where and with whom is your goal appropriate?
- What will you have to give up in order to get it?
- What will you see, hear and feel differently if you get it?
- What if you get it?
- Are you sure that you want it?
- Who else is involved?
- What resources do you have/do you need to move towards it?
- How will you know when you have it?
- What small step can be your first step, after answering these questions? (Knight, 2008)

If you have experienced SMART before, you will notice how these questions really add to your ability to think through a goal.

Time for reflection

How can knowledge of these things help you to build your career? Take a moment to think of a goal for your career. Run the idea through SMART, then the other questions, and then through SMART again. What you find easy and hard to answer suggests areas of strength and areas in need of development. Knowing what you want, and being able to articulate that, is attractive to potential employers. Being able to help others to set goals is a key management skill.

Money

Regardless of your moral imperative, you will need to be either directly responsible for, or contributing to, making money. Money comes into a business; a business spends money, so it goes out again. The trick lies in making sure that less goes out than comes in. Money coming into the business is simply *income*, money going out is *expenditure*, and this is the same regardless of the scale of the business. Keeping track on how much is coming in and going out is called *accounting*.

Income and expenditure

Money comes into businesses in various ways but the most simple is the transaction typified in the example of a client handing over cash to their chiropodist at the end of a treatment session. Other ways that the chiropodist can gain income are through winning a contract to provide services (e.g. to be the sole provider of chiropody care to all the residents in a retirement home), through selling chiropody equipment to clients at a price higher than the cost to the chiropodist, and through borrowing money from a bank. Each of these means of money coming into a business is known as an *income stream*. In principle, the more income streams, the safer a business is from damage to an income stream. The old adage, 'don't put all your eggs in one basket' holds true for business.

As businesses grow in complexity, so the income streams develop more complex processes in the name of fairness, governance, transparency, compliance, and so on. Regardless of the size of the business unit you are in (from sole trader to clinical manager of a clinical commissioning group in the UK NHS) it is worth keeping the simple description, given above, in mind. If you encounter a new piece of jargon, first clarify whether it refers to money coming in or going out of your business.

'Commissioning', 'purchasing', 'procurement', 'payment', 'investment', 'spend', 'cost': all these terms basically mean money flowing out of your business. Some are useful distinctions, others are merely euphemisms. Be mindful that as you engage with greater levels of complexity, the jargon intensifies, often due to the influence of business management culture rather than for practical clarity. Does the jargon term relate to 'money in' or 'money out'? Keep it simple. In an interview setting, you may feel tempted to join the jargon arms race but I recommend resisting that urge and, instead, talk in simple terms that really demonstrate your understanding, on a business level, of what the situation under discussion involves.

Accounting

If we pursue the metaphor of money flowing into a business in income streams then we can begin to understand the jargon term, 'cash flow'. The purpose of accounts is to record the money flowing into, and out of, your business.

Accounting is sometimes referred to as 'book keeping', which refers to the pre-technical era in which ledgers were used to record the accounts. Keeping one's books up to date is a vital need for any business in order to check the health of the business. If outflow out paces income then the business will have to depend upon an overdraft from its bank, or from loans from banks or investors, or face bankruptcy – the state of a business that cannot pay its debts.

Finance and accounting skills

Of course, you can pay for an accountant, but it is worth spending a little time to learn the accountant's language so that you will be able to understand their reports to you and that, even without the accountant's attention, you know how healthy your business is at any time. Even if you work as part of a business unit for which you have no direct accounting responsibility, some basic understanding will help you to appreciate the 'bottom line' and how your purchasing decisions are likely to affect the overall health of the business.

An essential, basic concept is 'cash flow'. Cash comes into the business through sales. It goes out of the business through purchases that the business makes. If not enough comes in to pay for the purchases (e.g. supplies, rent, rates, wages etc.) then the business will likely be declared bankrupt. The 'bottom line' is simply that which remains after all the expenses have been subtracted from the revenues (income minus expenditure or sales minus purchases). It is in the interest of the business to increase its bottom line. Notice that, yet again, it is possible to scale these concepts from the large corporation down to the individual. In other words, your personal income needs to exceed your personal expenditure or else you will face legal proceedings. The same applies to a business regardless of its size or its legal structure. Do remember, however, that the legal structure may offer the individual business owner some protection against personal loss should bankruptcy occur.

As mentioned, above, most large banks offer free business planning software with which you can learn some good habits of managing the finances of a business. Understanding what your business or business unit is spending versus what it is earning is essential to reduce waste, inform purchasing decisions and engender a sense of shared responsibility among the staff working in the business unit.

So what are 'accounts', and why bother? We bother with accounts in order to keep an eye on the bottom line and also because they are necessary as the basis of the government's tax calculations (personal tax and corporation tax). One of the expenses of a business is pay and the jargon for this tends to be, for a sole trader or partnership, 'drawings', and, for a limited company, salary or dividends. Keeping good accounts allows you to set your pay at a realistic level and to plan for developing this, if appropriate.

The accounts of a business are simply the detailed records of money in (sales) and money out (purchases). Of course, this quickly becomes more complicated and jargon-filled, but regardless of that complexity, it is worth remembering that business success depends upon money in remaining greater than money out. You will need to be aware of the means of credit – how to borrow money should your cash flow temporarily stop flowing in. For example, if a client is late in paying for a service that you have sold them and, as a consequence, you are unable to pay a supplier for materials that you need to buy, then you either have to cease trading (business) or borrow money to tide you over until the late payment is made. Again, an individual can use credit cards, have an overdraft with their bank, or take out a loan from their bank. Businesses basically do the same, though they may also raise money (get more into the business) by selling off assets, issuing more shares, or gain direct investment through, for example, venture capital (capital – cash – that is invested into a new or expanding business). Venture capital will never be gained to ease cash flow alone. Instead, it is seen as a type of gamble in which the payoff is a high return based on the improved business performance, measured by profit, of the business invested in.

Tax – income and corporation

All businesses, regardless of scale, pay tax. As a sole trader you will pay your own tax bill. Each director of a business pays their own tax independent of the company. A limited company pays Corporation Tax, as the business is considered a single entity paying its tax to the government. The same applies across most countries, but for a clear exposition of what taxes are required for different levels of business complexity Her Majesties Revenue & Customs office is a good place to look (www.hmrc.gov.uk). In the United Kingdom, other than income tax and corporation tax, knowledge of Value Added Tax (VAT) is necessary.

Tax – Value Added

Value Added Tax is a tax paid by customers to a business at each stage in the supply chain [Supply chain: take as an example, a bicycle. A business had to mine the metal ore and sell it to a metal foundry. That is two links in the supply chain. The foundry sells its metal to a manufacturer who makes bicycle frames but buys in the chains, brakes, saddles etc. necessary to make the finished bicycle. Each supplier to the manufacturer is another link in the chain. The manufacturer sells finished bicycles to bicycle shops: another link in the chain. Finally, the bicycle shop sells the bicycle to a customer]. At each stage in the supply chain each link pays VAT to the link that it bought supplies from. Each business in the supply chain have most of the VAT cost paid to its suppliers by the VAT paid to it when it sells on its products (the VAT paid to the manufacturers of bicycle chains will be mostly recovered by the VAT raised on the sale of the finished bicycle). Therefore, VAT raises money for the government at each stage of the supply chain but is ultimately paid by the final customer. Within the European Union, VAT is currently [2014] about 20%. In non-EU countries, most have some form of VAT, though this can range from zero (e.g. The British Caymen Islands, http://www.offtax.com/countries/cayman-islands/cayman-islands-tax-features.php) to 25.5% in Iceland (http://www.fita.org/countries/iceland.html).

It is worth noting that a business does not need to pay VAT in the United Kingdom until its turnover exceeds £81k/year (https://www.gov.uk/vat-registration). 'Turnover' is the same as 'revenue', that is, the income derived from the sale of goods and/or services that are the normal activities of the business.

Summary

Business: things, people, time and money. As you build your career in the health sector, try to keep the complex systems reduced to these simple terms. The more advanced a career becomes, the more complex the systems within which you move and, likely, attempt to control also become. Hold in mind as you observe a complex system, what the problems are; are they to do with 'things', people, time or money? If the problem is with 'things', is that the legal structure, or is it (more likely) to do with what you are spending your money on, or how money is coming into your business? If the problem is with 'people', is that an in-facing or out-facing problem, evidence of poor recruitment, a training need, or a disciplinary procedure? If the problem is with time, then that tends to suggest a staffing issue, a process issue or a training need. If the problem is to do with money, then that will be either money in or money out, or the relationship between them.

You do not need an MBA to run a business or business unit successfully, and do not be put off by the myriad models and processes found in business and management text books, and certainly do not be baffled or overawed by the worst type of 'management speak' that many texts and training programmes are in favour of.

Of course, there is always something to learn from those with more experience, but as you begin your career be mindful that you already have plenty of experience that you can articulate in ways to support your developing career.

Potential Interview questions in this area
- What entrepreneurial activity did you undertake during your degree?
- What relationships are there between your degree and business?
- Who are the stakeholders in your degree?

References

Blanchard K and Johnson S (2004) *The one minute manager*. New York: William Morrow and Company, Inc.

Cabinet Office (2010) *Building the big society*. Available at https://www.gov.uk/government/publications/building-the-big-society; last accessed 19 August 2015.

Covey SR (2004) *The 7 habits of highly successful people: Restoring the character ethic*. New York: Simon & Schuster, Inc.

Knight S (2008) *NLP at work: Neuro linguistic programming*, 2nd edn. London: Nicholas Brealey Publishing.

Luft J and Ingham H. (1955) *The Johari Window, a graphic model of interpersonal awareness*. Proceedings of the western training laboratory in group development, Los Angeles, CA: University of California, Los Angeles.

Rubin RS (2002) Will the real SMART goals please stand up? *The Industrial-Organizational Psychologist*, **39**(4):26–27 (http://www.siop.org/tip/backissues/TIPApr02/pdf/394_026to027.pdf; last accessed 12 August 2015).

Zeller D (2008) *Successful time management for dummies*. Hoboken: John Wiley & Sons, Inc.

Chapter 8 The job application process

Stephanie Allen

The Training Spa, Norwich, UK

This chapter seeks to set out the nuts and bolts of how to get your foot on the career ladder. It is written to be used as a very practical guide to support you in your job search now and throughout your career.

Getting behind the recruitment process

The decision to recruit is not a light undertaking. Organisations, whether in the public, private or third sector, will have put together a case to justify the extra spend involved in recruiting a new member of staff. This annual cost of salary and other expenses is in addition to the sometimes hidden cost of the recruitment process. It goes without saying, therefore, that employers need to recruit and retain the right person and will use a range of tools to ensure the process is effective.

What employers are looking for

In order to select fairly and get the right person for the job, employers follow a strict framework that sets out the skills, qualities and attributes required by the successful recruit. This framework forms the 'person specification' that will give you an insight into what is needed to gain the role. The skills, qualities and attributes are then defined as 'essential': in other words they are an absolute requirement, and 'desirable': good to have by the candidate. From a practical perspective, the organisation will require a transparent way of reducing the applications to a realistic number for interview. This means you have to prove that you possess all the essential criteria, if you are to stand a chance of gaining an interview. The most usual way of doing this is through production of your 'curriculum vitae' (CV) or 'story of life'.

How to Develop Your Healthcare Career: A Guide to Employability and Professional Development, First Edition. Edited by Lisa Taylor.
© 2016 John Wiley & Sons, Ltd. Published 2016 by John Wiley & Sons, Ltd.

Organisational sectors

Whether you are recent graduate or an experienced practitioner, you will see vacancies in all three sectors:

- public
- private
  - ◦ small and medium enterprises or SMEs (fewer than 249 employees)
  - ◦ large business (more than 250 employees)
- third (not-for profit or charity sector).

Whilst your CV will not look very different for each sector, it is worth taking time to consider the sector concerned. For example, public sector organisations will invariably be bigger, with set gradings for staff levels, and often more formalised in their practices. SMEs are, by definition, smaller and often less process driven. Large business may be 'corporates' that may have larger budgets and, therefore, higher pay scales. The third sector will include housing associations and similar and are very much values driven.

Your CV will be expected to reflect these differences to show your understanding of and to exhibit your commitment to the sector. Many organisations in all sectors will publish their values on their web site. It is worthwhile using the words of these in your CV as appropriate.

Job and person specifications

Any job advert will have attached to it a 'job description' and 'person specification'. The former sets out the role statement and responsibilities of the job. The latter identifies the skills, qualifications and attributes that are considered to be 'essential' and/or 'desirable' for the role. It is therefore important that your CV or application form shows, for every application, that you possess the 'essential' criteria and as many of the 'desirable' as possible.

Many organisations receive hundreds of applications and strive to be completely impartial and fair in how applicants are selected for interview. Only applicants possessing all the 'essential' criteria would normally be considered and if there are too many to interview, the number will be whittled down by measuring applicants against the 'desirable' criteria.

Introducing the CV

For many people this is a document that is written once and dusted off whenever a potential job comes into view. By definition, the CV is an up-to-date record of your skills and achievements. Therefore, it needs to be constantly updated and a true reflection of where you have been and where you are going. Perhaps even more importantly, it needs to reflect the skills, qualities and attributes required for each job application.

The Association of Graduate Recruiters (AGR) annual summer survey (http://www.bbc.co.uk/news/education-23247176) shows that leading UK employers are receiving an average of eighty five applications per job! In some sectors this increases to one hundred and fifty per job! This suggests that your CV must stand out and prove that you have all the 'essential' and as many of the 'desirable' criteria as possible.

Starting your CV

Trends in CV writing come and go, so it is important to stay up to date with current styles. The structure set out in this chapter is the generally accepted current model at time of publication.

Two key considerations must be borne in mind:

1. The CV is your selling document – your advert; but it should comply with the currently appreciated norms of CV writing. If it looks tired and out of date, or unprofessional in its spelling, layout and content, what does that say about you?
2. As much as many employers still manually sift applications to create a shortlist, an increasing number use electronic sifting software. This adds a new dimension to CV production, in that certain keywords from the person specification should be incorporated into your document. This is good practice in any situation, as it enables electronic or manual sifting to test the validity of the CV.

When you start your CV, it will be a brief framework of your study and any work to date. Once you start applying for jobs, it is important to consider how organisations define job roles and then use that information to 'flesh out' your CV.

CV layout

The key to an effective CV is to make it fit the role for which you are applying. This means each CV will be slightly different as you amend words and order to prove how you meet the essential criteria. We talk about 'white space'; in other words allow clear margins and good spacing so that whomever reads it, finds it easy to follow. With some managers only spending forty five seconds looking at each CV, you will need to make it as easy as possible! It is generally accepted that a CV should be no longer than two sides of A4 and use an internet-friendly font such as Times New Roman or Arial.

The currently accepted CV layout, for a recent graduate, covers the following in the order shown:

- personal details – name, address, telephone and email;
- a sentence or two, describing you, written in the third person:
  for example, a highly motivated, speech and language therapy graduate with a passion for research and practical problem solving. Confident communicator and presenter;
- your key skills, set out in bullet points, perhaps two or three together:
  for example, confident communicator with excellent presentation skills;

- education & training, in reverse chronological order;
- your experience, in reverse chronological order;
- other achievements;
- interests.

A sample CV layout suitable for a recent graduate is shown in Box 8.1.

Box 8.1 Sample CV for a recent graduate

Alison Barry
21 York Road, London SW14 2AB
0207 123 4567

alison.barry@gmail.com

Highly motivated and committed mature mental health nurse seeking a first post in inpatient care. Excellent team player with very strong communication skills. Seeking a position to build on experiences and make a valuable contribution to the nursing team.

Key Skills
- confident verbal communicator with excellent presentation skills
- able to build professional relationships at all levels
- effective organiser with excellent time management ability
- acquisitive desire to gain new skills & knowledge

Education
University of East Anglia – BSc in Nursing Studies (Mental Health) 2011–2014
Gained an insight into the demands of mental health nursing and worked as a member of the multidisciplinary team through undertaking placements in a range of clinical settings – acute, child & adolescent, forensic and elderly mentally ill. Developed skills in patient assessment, care planning, implementation and evaluation whilst working in consultation with clients and colleagues.

Honley High School, Huddersfield 2005–2011

6 GCSEs (Grades A–C) including Maths, English and Science.
3 A levels Biology, Sociology; Chemistry

Work Experience
Various clinical placements 2011–2014

June–September 2010 Brook Care Home, Huddersfield
                     – supported residents in a lively care environment
                     – worked in a shift-based team on a range of duties

Other achievements
Member of University sports committee, volunteer with the Prince's Trust.

Interests
I enjoy running for relaxation and run 5k races on a regular basis to raise money for Cancer Research UK.

If you have worked since graduating, the order changes thus:
- personal details;
- a sentence or two, describing you, written in the third person: for example, your key skills, set out in bullet points, perhaps two or three together;
- your experience, in reverse chronological order;
- education and training, in reverse chronological order;
- other achievements;
- interests.

Time for reflection

Consider your skills and experience to date. It's easy to dismiss the things you do as 'part of the job' or 'part of my course'. Employers are interested to learn 'how' you do things. They are keen to see appropriate behaviours. Your CPD portfolio is ideal for evidencing and recording relevant information.

Submitting your CV

Each application will require an amendment to your CV to change keywords. Add experience and achievements if appropriate, but also to ensure that the document is as fresh and relevant as possible.

Your CV needs a covering letter; something that augments the content of your CV with a specific focus on the job in question. The letter will be addressed to the named contact in the organisation. This may be 'Dear Jane Smith' or 'Dear Doctor Smith'. If unsure, telephone the organisation and ask how the person would prefer to be addressed. As you are writing to a named person, your signature would be prefixed by one of the following:
- yours sincerely (considered old-fashioned by many)
- best wishes
- kind regards.

Current thinking is that the term 'Dear sir or madam' is outmoded and should not be used. For that reason, the sign-off 'yours faithfully" is not appropriate either.

The letter offers you the opportunity to add value to your CV by stressing exactly how you are suited to the role in question and what you can bring to it. A sample letter is presented in Box 8.2.

Do not be tempted to use the e-mail text box in place of a separate letter. Your ability to set out a professional letter and CV tests written communication skills and it is vital that a letter format is maintained.

Box 8.2 Sample application covering letter

Sukhvinder Desai
58 Laburnam Close, London N14 2AB
0208 421 1234

sukhvinder@gmail.com

21/05/14

Dear Jane Smith

I am delighted to attach my CV for the post of Mental Health Guidance Worker as advertised on your website. I have been interested in the work of 'Mind' for many years as I have seen the practical outcomes you offered to a close friend.

As you will see from my attached CV, I am a recent graduate with a passion for working within the mental health profession. My degree offered a host of opportunities which I grasped fully to build a broad portfolio of skills and knowledge and am keen to work alongside young people through their challenges and opportunities.

Throughout my studies I have learnt resilience and considerable self-awareness; two qualities that I know will support my skills and my interactions with others.

I very much hope that I will be able to discuss this further with you at interview.

Best wishes

Sukhvinder Desai

Here are ten tips for the perfect CV:

1. Do not put 'CV' or 'curriculum vitae' at the top!
2. Refrain from using headings such as 'name' or 'address'!
3. Use a reader-friendly font such as Arial or Times New Roman.
4. Keep it concise, normally within two pages.
5. Check spelling and check again.
6. Do not include irrelevant information such as marital status, date of birth or number of children.
7. Use the words and language from the person specification.
8. Offer examples to prove the skills you have.
9. Focus on your achievements. Show HOW you have done something rather than WHAT you have done.
10. *Never lie* about your qualifications or experience.

What can go wrong

Employers often have to sift through a vast number of CVs and will quickly reject those that are difficult to read or miss out important information. When asked by the largest online recruiter, Careerbuilder (www.careerbuilder. co.uk), what makes employers reject candidates, the results make interesting reading. CVs are invariably rejected if they:

- have spelling mistakes or typos (61%);
- use large amounts of wording from the job posting (41%);
- show an inappropriate e-mail address (35%);
- do not include a list of skills (30%);
- are more than two pages long (22%);
- are printed on decorative paper (20%);
- detail more tasks than results for previous positions (16%);
- include a photo (13%);
- have large blocks of text with little white space (13%).

Other application processes

Whilst the CV is considered the most effective way of sharing your skills and experience with potential employers, it is not the only method used by organisations to recruit people. There is an argument that using CVs could lead to inconsistency in the process and that employers may subconsciously discriminate (for example, a negative view might be taken if your CV is not in the latest style!). In order to prevent this, organisations may have very specific processes for gaining applications:

- application forms
- application forms plus CV
- online application processes.

Whichever method is used by your potential employer, your CV will give you the information required and is, therefore, a great guide to completing other types of application.

When completing a printed or online application form, it is appropriate to use the wording and content of your CV, but make sure you are fulfilling the requests of the form.

Many public sector organisations, including the NHS, have their own online processes. These are often very prescriptive but invariably include detailed guidance.

The personal statement

Many application forms offer space for your 'personal statement'; your opportunity to flesh out the bland content of the form. Leap at this chance to sell yourself! You may be limited to one side of A4, so maximise your precise skills and remove the temptation to start all your sentences with the pronoun 'I' by using headings (taken from the job and person specifications) with bullet points. For example, a person specification with the essential criterion 'able to work within a team' might be reflected in your personal statement thus:

Ability to work within a team

• *thrived on recent experiences in a small team of five, working on a change project; was keen to learn from other team members as well as offering support in my specialist field*

Your personal statement, as in your CV, should be easy to read – lots of white space!

Time for reflection

Application complete! In the time between submitting your application and gaining an interview, consider how you will research the organisation and the role. Take time to research more broadly within the sector concerned. What do you know about the bigger picture?

Preparing for the interview

Let us assume that your focused CV has been submitted and you receive an invitation to interview. Your natural excitement should be tempered by the preparation process needed to be successful.

Initial preparation

Whilst the interview is still used by many organisations as the sole method of selection, there is a growing trend to use a range of assessment methods. The reasoning behind this is that an interview, often only forty or so minutes, does not allow the potential employer to see candidates 'in action'. For example, a common key requirement is to be able to 'work in a team'. The interviewer can encourage the applicant to give examples of when he or she worked in a team but it does not truly test this in a real-life situation.

The use of 'assessment centres', where all the shortlisted candidates participate in one or more activities designed around the key requirements of the person specification, offers a much more realistic test of skills, qualities and attributes. An assessment centre can include:

• team activities or tests, where all candidates are observed whilst fulfilling a task or activity;

• aptitude tests on specific skills, such as information technology (IT), literacy or numeracy;

- presentations, where the applicant is asked to plan and deliver a presentation about a pre-determined topic;
- psychometric testing or profiling; the former indicates how good someone is at a particular skill, such as verbal or numerical reasoning and the latter 'builds a picture' of the candidate by identifying their values, personality type or occupational interests.

The invitation to interview should indicate whether the process will be 'just' an interview, or if other forms of assessment will be used. If this information is not offered, it would be beneficial to contact the organisation and ask.

The interview itself

From the day you are invited, until you leave the interview room, your focus will be on the impression you make in your appearance, behaviour, attitude and communication skills. The preparation you put in will reap huge benefits.

Logistics

Where is the interview being held? Do you know how to get there? Can you ensure you arrive at the right time!

It might seem unnecessary to even ask these questions, but you will need to arrive around fifteen minutes before your allotted time, in order to gain composure and feel raring to go. Getting lost, being unable to park and missing your train are all guaranteed to ruin your interview. Research the location; check the best method of transport and allow plenty of time for hold-ups.

Building knowledge

Employers expect you to prove that you really want to work for them; that they are not one of many you have applied to and that you will just take the first offer. Your proof will be in your knowledge of the organisation.

Research as much as you can about the organisation. The person specification will guide you in thinking more deeply about the job and how you might apply your skills in context. Research more widely about the sector so that you can position the organisation more effectively. If you have been told who will be on the interview panel, find out about them. The business networking site LinkedIn (www.linkedin.com) will help here.

You will find it less stressful if you have considered the possible questions that you might be asked. The majority of interviewers use 'competency-based questions'. These enable you to give examples of how you use the skills and behaviours asked for in the person specification. For example, if an essential requirement is 'the ability to work in a team', the resulting competency based question might be:

'Tell me about your experiences as a team worker.'

or

'Tell me about a time you joined a team; how did you get to know your colleagues?'

Consider the questions that might come from each 'essential' or 'desirable' criterion and practice (perhaps in front of a mirror, or with someone) a range of answers.

Building interview skills

How you answer questions is not just about the validity of the words you use. The way we say something is just as, if not more, important. Research by Albert Mehabrian (1972), suggests that the messages we transmit are received as follows:

- 7% understanding through our spoken words;
- 38% through our voice, tone, eye contact, pitch and so on (paralinguistics);
- 55% via general body language and gestures.

It goes without saying, therefore, that in your responses you should match the words with your body language and tone!

At the end of every interview, the interviewers invariably invite you to ask any questions you have. It would not be a good move to ask about salary or bonuses but it is worth preparing two or three questions that would show you have thought about the process. Remember that a job interview is a two-way process. You are investigating whether you want to work for the organisation concerned just as much as the organisation is testing you, as already discussed in Chapter 1. It might be useful to jot your questions into a notebook or onto your phone or tablet.

Your image

You never get a second chance to make a first impression!

Dressing for the interview is often perceived as difficult. Rightly or wrongly, we are judged (often subconsciously) on our appearance. Think of your own response to people and what they wear. For job interviews, there is the dilemma of being yourself, yet appearing appropriately dressed for the interviewers.

If you can research the usual dress of the organisation, then you have a starting point. Yet, whilst dressing to 'fit' into the culture of the organisation, there is a sense that you still need to portray an image that meets the expectations of the interviewing panel. It is worth considering the basic rules:

- Men – a suit is not always necessary but smart trousers, shirt and jacket are. Wear shoes not trainers.

• Women – smart clothes, not too short or low cut, not too much jewellery. Smart shoes.

Preparing for an assessment centre

Once you know that there is any form of testing, then you can practice!

Psychometric tests are available online and, as well as giving you the chance to become familiar with the concept, will enable you to learn a great deal about yourself. With psychometric tests, there are no right or wrong answers; just a view about you and your thought process or personality.

Your invitation to interview might ask you to give a presentation. If so, consider carefully the brief and be particularly aware of the time constraint given. Naturally, you will make sure that any technology you use is compatible with the equipment offered. The ability to give a presentation is a good test of your communication skills, your ability to translate information into easily understood messages and your skill at not relying on technology! Please do not rely on IT-based programmes to do the work for you.

Consider what you know about any activities. Will you be working with other candidates? If so, how do you want to be seen? As a leader? A follower? Someone who pulls their weight? Someone who listens? Someone who communicates confidently but sensitively? Activities will be observed and how you respond will give the observers a view of you that may influence the interview. In some situations, an observed activity may be used as a way to eliminate candidates before the interview!

In the interview room

With the right preparation, you will arrive at the interview venue with time to spare. Arriving about 15 minutes before the appointment is considered appropriate. Time to relax, calm down and get focused on the next hour or so. Your image is also portrayed by your attitude. Walking confidently into the interview room (yes, you will feel nervous, but nobody else sees that!), offering a firm handshake, smiling and making eye contact all add to the overall impression.

When you are offered a seat, feel free to move it slightly, perhaps at a slight angle to the interviewers, so that you are not face-on (which can feel confrontational) and to allow you to take control of your space!

Handling questions

Thinking back to your preparation, you will have some idea of the questions asked. It is important to listen carefully, without interrupting the interviewer. Take a few seconds to consider your answer and then, making eye contact and alert to your tone and gestures, make your response.

Potential interview questions in this area
- Tell me about a time you had to confront a difficult situation?
- Describe a situation where you had to work as part of a team. What were the team's aims? What were the challenges?
- Please give an example of a time where you developed working relationships with people from different backgrounds. What skills did you use?

For each of these, and similar questions, your preparation will come into its own. Remember to answer concisely but with the detail required and without veering off-course!

At the end of the interview, when you are asked, 'Do you have any questions for us?'; you can refer to your prepared questions and ask.

Once the interview is over, rise from your seat, smile at the interviewer or panel, thank them for their time and stride confidently out of the room.

Time for reflection

Interviews are two way! It is very easy to only focus on the fact that employer is testing you. The interview is your chance to test out whether you want to work for the organisation concerned, so research thoroughly before you attend and think carefully of questions that you can ask to help you decide if you wish to take up the post!

What next?

Let us assume that you are offered the job, well done! If not, however, it is vital to learn from the experience and ask for feedback. Some organisations give feedback to everyone but with others you need to ask. Feedback is a great opportunity to learn and to put new ideas into practice.

A useful checklist to help with the interview process is given in Box 8.3.

Box 8.3 A checklist for the interview process

Interviews
- Plan for the interview
- Where is it? (It goes without saying that you need to check the location of the interview!)
- How do I get there? How long is the journey?
- How long will the interview take?

- What format will it take? (Assessment centres? Psychometric tests? Presentation? Aptitude test?)
- Who will interview me?
- Do I need to take certificates and so on?
- Assessment centres – an important opportunity to prove yourself
- What are your aims? (Interviews are as much about checking out if you want the job as much as about the employer wanting you)

Interview skills coaching
- Practise, practise, practise
- Assessment centres practice
- Self-assessment

Interview preparation
- Link the job description and person specification to your preparation process – understand the words used and deciding how to use them
- You never get a second chance..., clothes, making an entry
- Verbal, non-verbal and paralinguistics
- Competency-based questions – think of evidence
- Assessment centres – behaviours
- 'Do you have any questions for us?' Yes you do!! You have written them in a notebook or on your tablet – refer to them to show you are prepared!

The results!
- Good news!
- Not so good news – seek feedback
- What to do differently next time

Reference

Mehrabian A (1972) *Nonverbal communication*. Chicago, IL: Aldine-Atherton.

Further reading

Billsberry J (2000) *Finding and keeping the right people*, 2nd edn. London: Prentice-Hall.
Cowling A and Mailer C (1981) *Managing human resources*. London: Edward Arnold.
Ludlow R and Panton F (1991) *The essence of successful staff selection*. London: Prentice-Hall.

Chapter 9 Consolidation of learning and moving forward

This book has provided you with a wealth of information on aspects of employability that are relevant to healthcare students/graduates, wherever you decide to work. There have been questions posed throughout the book to encourage your personal reflection whilst reading each chapter. This final chapter offers you the main learning points from each chapter and the chance to consolidate your learning through a number of specific activities related to each chapter. This information can be used as evidence for your continuing professional development, which is essential to maximise your learning (Hong and Harrison, 2012, p. 9) and will build your confidence in articulating and further action planning your own employability journey.

The following activity is relevant and can be applied to all of the chapters that you have read in this book:

Develop an action plan on how are you going to implement the knowledge gained through each chapter into your own employability journey.

• What have you learned during this chapter?
• What are the key things that you want to work on from this chapter?
• Why are these key things important to you in your journey of employability?
• How are you going to implement your learning into your daily life?
• Who is going to be needed to help you implement your learning?
• When are you going to undertake this activity?

How to Develop Your Healthcare Career: A Guide to Employability and Professional Development, First Edition. Edited by Lisa Taylor.
© 2016 John Wiley & Sons, Ltd. Published 2016 by John Wiley & Sons, Ltd.

Chapter 1 – What is employability and what does it mean for you?

Key learning points

1. Employability is a lifelong journey.
2. A number of models exist for employability to frame your own employability journey.
3. Evidencing your employability is crucial for potential employment opportunities.

Activity – What is your approach to employability?

Are you happy with developing your existing strengths around employability or do you have an aspirational approach to employability – aspiring to achieve stronger levels of employability in your areas of weakness? Carry out an analysis on your personal development towards employability – what are your strengths and weaknesses?

Chapter 2 – Career planning and management

Key learning points

1. There are many ways to explore your career, and using different tools and perspectives can be helpful.
2. Your career is influenced by a range of external factors, some of which you have more control over than others.
3. You career trajectory is unlikely to be straightforward and may be a very odd 'shape'.

Activity 1 – Personal values and motivators exercise

In the follow exercise, think about what motivates you and whether the statements you choose are reflected in the career decisions you have made so far and are thinking of for the future.

Your values will change over time. For example, you may not feel limited by caring responsibilities at the moment but this may change as you become a parent or family members age? You may not yet realise the importance of exercising knowledge and becoming 'expert' in something, as you are still gaining in knowledge and confidence.

You may like to score these values on a scale of 1–10, and consider the highest and lowest scoring: are you surprised at the values that score most highly? Are they values that are common to your work? Are there values that contradict your work?

How do I want to work?
I want the *autonomy* to have the freedom to define my own work
I want *independence* to make some of my own decisions
I want to be *challenged* and be expected to work under pressure
I want to be *physically challenged* in my work
I want to be able to *take risks* and be adventurous
I want to work in a role that is *clearly structured* and has boundaries
I want to work in a way that reflects my spiritual or religious beliefs
I want to be at the cutting edge in my field

Why do I want to work?
I want to contribute to *helping society*
I want to *help others* and make a difference to people's day-to-day lives
I want to make a *difference to my organisation* and drive it forward
I want to *earn* a lot of money
I want to be in a position to *change the attitudes of others*
I want to bring my *knowledge and intellect* to bear on my work

Where do I want to work?
I want to be in a supportive environment where *helping others* is at the heart
I want to be in a **diverse environment**
I want to be in a place where *environmental values* are important
I want to be in a place that is *exciting* and always stimulating
I want to be in a place that has a clear *structure and processes*
I want to be in a place where I feel *valued* and I get feedback for my work

Who do I want to work with?
I want to work as an equal as part of a *team*
I want to work collaboratively and *sharing common goals* is important to me
I want to have responsibility for *managing others*
I want to work with people who are like me and *share my values*
I want to work in a place that is *friendly and fun*

What do I want to achieve?
I want *status* and the opportunity to move through the organisation
I want to be allowed to *specialise* and become expert in my field
I want to be able to *earn well*
I want *stability* and a clear career structure
I want to be challenged and expected to keep *learning*

Where do I want to be?
I want to remain close to *family and friends*
I want to be in a place where I can find a good *work-life balance*
I want to be part of a wider *community*
I want to work in a way that lets me *travel* and experience new places and
organisations
Others of your own?

Activity 2 – Attributes

Attributes are more innate than skills: they are about who you are, rather than what you do. Whilst we can develop attributes and use them to support our skills, working 'against type' can make our working life challenging; working 'to type' allows us to play to our strengths.

Shown in the next table are words you might use to describe yourself or that others might use to describe you.

Which of these attributes do you think sum you up?

Circle the ones that you think apply the most and then consider the questions following the table.

Try to think of **examples**, particularly for attributes that you initially think you might lack.

Are you sure? How might others describe you? Would they think of examples that you might overlook? Remember – you need to be fair on yourself in order to get a clear picture.

Accurate	Open-minded	Diplomatic	Responsible
Adaptable	Optimistic	Discreet	Risk-taking
Ambitious	Organized	Easy-going	Self-confident
Analytical	Patient	Efficient	Sensitive
Assertive	Persevering	Empathetic	Sociable
Calm	Persuasive	Enthusiastic	Supportive
Cautious	Practical	Kind	Tactful
Clear-thinking	Realistic	Logical	Tenacious
Conscientious	Reflective	Loyal	Thorough
Conservative	Reliable	Mature	Trusting
Creative	Reserved	Methodical	Trustworthy
Curious	Resourceful	Meticulous	Understanding
		Modest	Witty

- How have they helped you in your career to date?
- Have you experienced working environments where some/all of these attributes have been supported and used?
  - Conversely, have you worked in a place where they were suppressed? How does this affect your work?
- Think about those listed that you do not associate with yourself. Are there attributes that you think you need to practise in the future? Are there things that perhaps hold you back?

Chapter 3 – Professionalism

This chapter looked at professionalism from a sociological perspective.

Key learning points

1. To explain how professions are organised.
2. To define the concept of professionalism.
3. To describe how professionalism may be evidenced.

Try this reflective task to develop insights about your professionalism.

Activity

Look at professional responsibilities outlined in Table 3.1. Think about what each of them means to you and how you would provide evidence for each responsibility.

How can you enhance any responsibilities that need work?

For example, if you wanted to consider 'Personal Accountability' you might want to reflect on your engagement with social media. You could read the following articles:

Cunningham A (2014) Social media and medical professionalism. *Medical Education*, **48**:110–112.

Kleebauer A (2014) When trouble can be just a click away. *Nursing Standard*, **28**(49):20–21.

Osman A, Wardle A and Caesar R (2012) Online professionalism and Facebook – Falling through the generation gap. *Medical Teacher*, **34**:e549–e556.

Reed D, Mueller PS, Hafferty FW and Brennan MD (2013) Contemporary issues in medical professionalism. Challenges and opportunities. *Minnesota Medicine*, **96**(11):44–47.

Having done this you could consider:
- Am I being responsible enough when using Facebook?
- Am I risking too much disclosure about my clients?
- How is my professional presentation reflected in my postings?
- Am I maintaining appropriate boundaries with my clients?

You could write a reflective account. Then you have a piece of evidence that covers four of the responsibilities under the concept of professional accountability.

Chapter 4 – Continuing professional development

Key learning points

1. CPD is a fundamental part of delivering safe and effective patient care, and developing a meaningful and satisfying health and social care career.
2. CPD is a key pillar of employability. It should be a systematic process of identifying your learning needs, considering effective ways to conduct your learning, applying your learning to practice, evidencing your learning and utilising CPD to help build the career you want.

3. Whilst it is essential to be aware of your regulatory body's requirements around CPD for reregistration and/or revalidation, CPD is far more than a tick box exercise.

Activity 1

A PESTEL analysis is a simple tool used to analyse how various external factors may impact on the future. The P in PESTEL stands for political factors, E for economic factors, S for sociological factors, T for technological factors, E for environmental factors and L for legal factors. Take a moment to look up PESTEL on an Internet search engine.

Use the PESTEL framework to consider which factors are likely to impact on the next 5–10 years of your career in health and care.

For example: political factors may include older voters becoming more significant as the population ages; economic factors could include taxes on sugary foods or increased debt amongst graduates; sociological factors could include global migration or health inequalities between rich and poor; technological factors may include genomic sequencing, so everyone has access to their own genetic sequence, or wearable devices that capture parameters, such as weight or blood pressure, on a daily basis; environmental factors may include greater air pollution in cities or more intensive farming to feed a growing global population; legal factors could include increased health-related litigation.

Activity 2

In your field of interest set out to identify at least two of each of the following organisations/individuals who provide CPD in your area:
• CPD leads in your placement / employing organisation
• Publishers
• Learned societies
• LinkedIn groups
• Twitter streams
• Expert blogs
• UK universities and international universities.

Activity 3

Go online to your regulatory body. Follow the links to their CPD pages. Carefully consider how your regulatory body advises that your record your CPD activity. *Do they require you to keep a portfolio? What types of information must you to keep? How do they suggest you keep this information? (e.g. e-portfolio, paper record).*

Chapter 5 – Leadership

Key learning points

1. Good leadership is essential to high quality, safe patient care.
2. Leadership skills and behaviours can be learnt, practiced and improved but they are always personal.
3. Leadership is an essential component of your employability portfolio.

Activity – What is your approach to leadership?

Reflecting on this chapter, what personal characteristics do you have now which will help you develop as a leader? What do you consider to be your areas for development?

Chapter 6 – Service improvement

Key learning points

1. Service improvement requires problem solving skills. You will be able to use your experiences to demonstrate how you have assessed your service, identified the root cause of a problem and made suggestions for improvement.
2. Service improvement requires team work. You will be able to use your experiences to demonstrate how you have worked with others to achieve a shared goal of improving the quality of your service.
3. Service improvement requires creative and innovative thinking. You will be able to use your experiences to demonstrate how you have viewed change as an opportunity to improve quality, whilst making best use of resources.

Activity – Reflecting on your service improvement experience and transferrable skills for employment

Familiarise yourself with Core Dimension 4 of the Knowledge and Skills Framework for Health (KSF) (http://www.nhsemployers.org/PayAndContracts/AgendaForChange/KSF/Simplified-KSF/Pages/SimplifiedKSF.aspx)

Core Dimension 4 – Service Improvement:

- Level 1: Make changes in own practice and offer suggestions for improving services.
- Level 2: Contribute to the improvement of services.
- Level 3: Appraise, interpret and apply suggestions, recommendations and directives to improve services.
- Level 4: Work in partnership with others to develop, take forward and evaluate direction, policies and strategies.

Identify examples from your experience that you can use as evidence to support your achievements at levels 1, 2 and, if possible, level 3. Practice articulating these so that you can explain yourself clearly and logically in an interview situation.

Consider ways that you could demonstrate leadership potential by showing an awareness of how you might be able contribute to activities at level 4 in the future.

Chapter 7 – Business skills

Key learning points

1. Business is essentially simple. Regardless of the complexity of the business infrastructure, all businesses can be reduced to Things, People, Time and Money.

2. Know who you need to pay attention to. The bigger the business, the greater the number of stakeholders, some of whom are to do with operating the business (in-facing) and others to do with external constraints, such as policy, and markets and customers (out-facing). Where you put your attention is vital.

3. Money flows into the business, money flows out. Again, regardless of the size of the business this holds true, so be mindful of that. If you are spending money, where is it coming from? Where is it going to? How does money flow into the business?

Activity

- Review some aspect of your life, so far, and identify a business with which you are familiar. Identify the goods or services sold, the legal structure, the stakeholders, the business goals and strategies, and what you can about the financial dealings of the business.

- Use a business plan template to set out your findings in (this is excellent practise for you to learn to articulate ideas in a business discourse, and this can be impressive to potential employers).

- Create a business plan for some imagined small business or business unit that you are genuinely interested in. If you wish to work in a large public organisation, remember to approach it through the simple headings of this chapter. Use the same business plan template and see how far you can go.

Business planning software is freely available from all high street banks. However, you may like to investigate these business planning templates, all of which are free at this time (November 2014):

- http://www.sage.co.uk/business-advice/starting-a-business/guide-starting-a-business.html?nst=0&gclid=CM2p_Z27yMICFSX4wgod-UYAJQ#

- https://www.gov.uk/write-business-plan
- http://nhshealthatwork.co.uk/business-plan-resources.asp

Chapter 8 – The job application process

Key learning points

1. Your CV is your marketing document.
2. Each time you submit a CV or application form, it should evidence the requirements of the person specification.
3. Interviews require lots of planning and preparation!
4. Interviews are your opportunity to shine and to prove your worth to a potential employer, but are also your chance to see if you want to work for the organisation concerned.

Activity

Having considered the value of a CV, think about the skills you have gained over your life. List them and then arrange them in two or three word phrases. For example your skills might include:

- getting on with people
- face to face communication
- IT skills
- giving presentations
- team working
- project management.

These could be grouped in the 'key skills' section of your CV as follows:

- Confident communicator with a dynamic presentation style.
- Motivational team worker, experienced in managing projects.

Write down your key skills.

How would you design your opening statement? Can you define you and your style in one or two sentences?

Thinking about job interviews, what questions would you want to ask a potential employer to show that you are serious about the role?

Activity

Access a job description and personal specification for a job that may be of interest for you to apply for within the next six months. Write down how you would evidence that you fulfil aspects of the job description and personal specification. Make a note on what you need to work and develop an action plan to be able to work towards fulfilling all aspects of the job description and personal specification in the coming months.

Consolidation of learning and moving forward conclusions

Having worked through the activities for all of the chapters you should have consolidated your employability-related knowledge learned through reading this book. You will also have generated a number of valuable resources to add to your continuing professional development portfolio. Having worked through the activities you should now be able to confidently articulate and evidence your knowledge and experience in employability related factors. You should also be able to further action plan your future employability development as part of your continuous life journey, wherever you are planning to work.

Reference

Hong and Harrison (2012) *Tools for continuing professional development.* 2nd edn. London: Quay Books, MA Healthcare Limited.

Index

How to Develop Your Healthcare Career: A Guide to Employability and Professional Development, First Edition. Edited by Lisa Taylor.
© 2016 John Wiley & Sons, Ltd. Published 2016 by John Wiley & Sons, Ltd.